4/20

$34.95
B/DRAKE
Diller, Philip M.
Leaving a legacy

D1260010

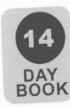

14
DAY
BOOK

LEAVING A LEGACY

LEAVING A LEGACY

Lessons *from the Writings of*
Daniel Drake

Philip M. Diller, MD, PhD

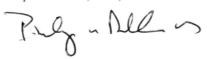

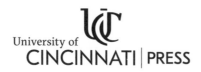

University of
CINCINNATI | PRESS

About the University of Cincinnati Press
The University of Cincinnati Press is committed to publishing rigorous, peer reviewed, leading scholarship accessibly to stimulate dialog between the academy, public intellectuals and lay practitioners. The Press endeavors to erase disciplinary boundaries in order to cast fresh light on common problems in our global community. Building on the university's longstanding tradition of social responsibility to the citizens of Cincinnati, state of Ohio, and the world, the press publishes books on topics which expose and resolve disparities at every level of society and have local, national and global impact.

The University of Cincinnati Press, Cincinnati 45221
Copyright © 2019

ISBN 978-1-947602-42-7 (hardback)
ISBN 978-1-947602-44-1 (e-book, PDF)
ISBN 978-1-947602-43-4 (e-book, EPUB)

Library of Congress Cataloging-in-Publication Data

Diller, Philip M., author.
Leaving a legacy : lessons from the writings of Daniel Drake / Philip M. Diller, MD.
Cincinnati, Ohio : University of Cincinnati Press, 2019. |
    Includes bibliographical references.
LCCN 2018059033| ISBN 9781947602427 (hardback) | ISBN
    9781947602441 (ebook, pdf) | ISBN 9781947602434 (e-book, epub)
LCSH: Drake, Daniel, 1785-1852--Health. | Medical
    writing--History--19th century. | Physicians--United States. | BISAC:
    MEDICAL / Education & Training. | MEDICAL / Essays.
LCC R119 .D55 2019 | DDC 808.06/661--dc23 LC record available at https://lccn.loc.gov/2018059033

Designed and produced for UC Press by Orange Frazer Press, Wilmington, Ohio
Typeset in: Wilmington, Ohio
Printed in the United States of America

First Printing

Dedication

This book is dedicated to my formative teachers, Paul Homer and Richard Bell, who introduced me to the human character and its place in the affairs of man, to Godfrey Getz, who taught me persistence in the pursuit of truth and excellence, and to Robert Smith, who modeled his passion for academic medicine and literature.

"It would be premature to predict what estimate will be placed upon Drake's works by posterity.... Truth is eternal, and whatever of this sublime essence his works contain must be transmitted from one generation to another so long as man remains a civilized being, and possesses the faculty of communicating knowledge. Based as they are on upon the observation of nature, and the just interpretation of her laws, they must always remain an ever-green beauty and freshness.... The student will always find in them a never-failing source of instruction and enjoyment."

—Samuel D. Gross.

"A Discourse on the Life, Character, and Services of Daniel Drake, MD."
Delivered before the faculty and the medical students of the University of Louisville, January 27, 1853.
Louisville: *The Louisville Journal,* 1853

Contents

❖

FOREWORD
by Andrew Filak *page xi*

EPITAPHS
page xiii

INTRODUCTION
Creating a Legacy *page xvii*

1. MAN
The Formative Influences That
Shaped Drake as a Person *page 3*

2. CITIZEN
How Drake Impacted His
Community to Build and Shape an
Advancing Culture *page 47*

3. WRITER
Finding a Voice and Style to Frame
and Influence *page 104*

4. EDUCATOR
Being an Innovator and Setting High
Standards for Education *page 157*

5. PHYSICIAN
A Master Physician with a Broad
Understanding of the Patient and
Practice *page 194*

EPILOGUE
Drake's Legacy Today *page 251*

DANIEL DRAKE CHRONOLOGY
October 20, 1785–November 5, 1852
page 255

ACKNOWLEDGMENTS
page 263

CITED WRITINGS OF DANIEL DRAKE
page 267

Foreword

The legacy of Daniel Drake has had a tremendous impact on the University of Cincinnati and the entire greater Cincinnati region. His creation of the Medical College of Ohio, with its charter issued in 1819, provided the foundation for what has evolved into the University of Cincinnati. The University and its College of Medicine have long and storied histories. As we celebrate our bicentennial it is fitting that Philip Diller, MD, PhD, offers his reflections on the life and work of a founder, Daniel Drake. It is also fitting, as we enter our bicentennial year, to note that the strategic direction of Next Lives Here with its platforms of Academic Excellence, Urban Impact, and Innovation Agenda are fully in line with Drake's original vision.

Daniel Drake, MD, who has been referred to as "the Benjamin Franklin of the West," combined an extraordinary medical career with unparalleled contributions in education, science, literature, and civic engagement. As Dr. Diller notes, education was critical to Drake's personal development and to the development of a vital community culture. He outlines here Drake's accomplishments as a man, a citizen, a writer, a teacher, and a physician. Particularly pertinent to our current day and age is the concept that life's random events call for a response or an opportunity to assume responsibility or not. It is ever clear that Drake chose the opportunities to assume responsibility. He responded to tragedies such as the death of his wife, children, father, and cousin with a resolve and a sense of purpose and was truly transformative with his words and in his actions.

In 1985, in celebration of the two hundredth anniversary of the birth of its founder, the College of Medicine established the Daniel Drake Medal, the highest honor bestowed upon living faculty and alumni. Those chosen for this award have followed in Drake's footsteps with their contributions and achievements. As noted by Charles Aring, MD, who was one of the first recipients of the Drake Medal, in his 1985 article in the *Journal of the American Medical Association*, "For William Osler,

Daniel Drake was a unique figure in American medicine and the founder of nearly everything that is old and good in Cincinnati."

Dr. Diller provides us the opportunity to reflect upon the contributions of Daniel Drake. He offers us the ability to see Drake not only through Drake's writings but also those of Diller, who has become a student of this innovative, creative, and complex man. There are many lessons to be learned from Drake. I am particularly struck by the sense of the transformative power of an individual, the resilience in the face of adversity and using adversity as an opportunity to assume responsibility to move forward, and the overall need for a sense of purpose. And this book provides us the opportunity for reflection. Reflection on the contributions of Daniel Drake. Reflections on our past as a medical school, as a university, and as a city. And in reflecting on our past, Diller expresses the opportunity to move forward following the legacy of Dr. Drake: "A legacy that others value can result from acts emanating from great character, being a servant who offers a helping hand, using power to do good, improving and building community, educating and providing wise counsel, defining and shaping a field of endeavor, or creating technological innovations—all to benefit the lives of others."

—Andrew Filak

Interim Senior Vice President for Health Affairs

and Dean of the College of Medicine

University of Cincinnati

Epitaphs

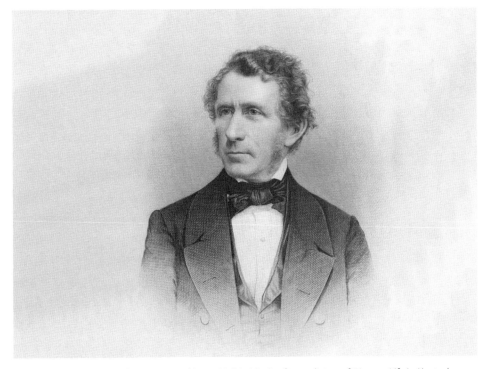

Daniel Drake, aet. sixty-five, engraved by A. H. Ritchie for first edition of *Pioneer Life in Kentucky*.

"Sacred to the Memory of Daniel Drake, a learned and distinguished physician, an able and philosophic writer, an eminent teacher of the medical art, a citizen of exemplary virtue and public spirit, a man rarely equaled in all the gentler qualities which adorn social and domestic life. His fame is indelibly written in the records of his country. His good deeds, impressed on beneficent public institutions, endure forever. He lived in the fear of God and died in the hope of salvation. He who lies here was an early inhabitant and untiring friend of the City of Cincinnati with whose prosperity his fame is inseparably connected."

— Words on Daniel Drake's Spring Grove Cemetery Monument

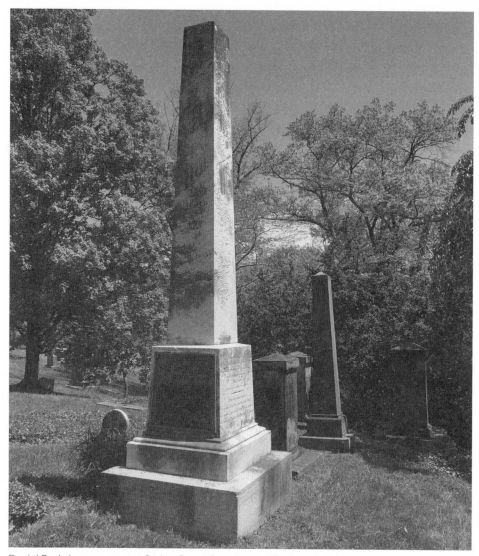

Daniel Drake's monument at Spring Grove Cemetery in Cincinnati, Ohio. *Photo by the author.*

"Resolved: That his steady devotion to his profession through a long life, and his zeal, activity, and unceasing efforts to advance its interest, afford an example worthy of imitation of every young physician.

Resolved: That this Association will cherish the memory of Dr. Drake for his many virtues, and for his labors, which have adorned and elevated our profession."

— American Medical Association, *Transactions* 6 (1853): 42

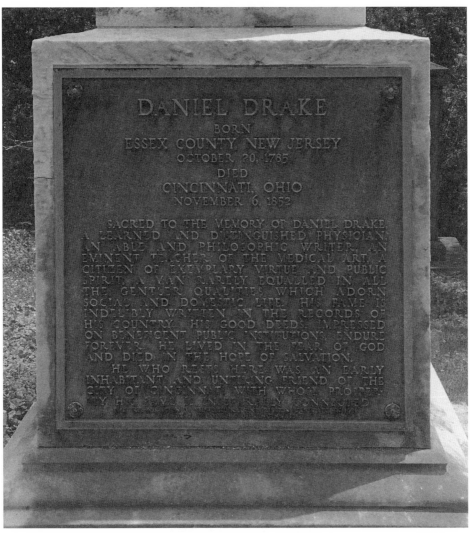

Bronze plaque reproducing the original inscription carved into Drake's monument; placed by Cincinnati physicians in 1952. *Photo by the author.*

"So many good works did he undertake, so much did he accomplish, so effectually did he stimulate exertion in others, both friends and enemies, that I think he may be called with propriety the *Franklin of Cincinnati.*"

—W. H. Venable, *Beginnings of Literary Culture in the Ohio Valley, Historical and Biographical Sketches* (Cincinnati: Robert Clarke & Co., 1891), 304.

Introduction

✠ CREATING A LEGACY

In 1850, the American Medical Association, only four years old at the time, met in Cincinnati. At the meeting Dr. Alfred Stille, of Philadelphia, reviewed notable medical works and gave lavish praise to Daniel Drake's recent publication, the first volume of *The Diseases of the Interior Valley of North America*, referring to it as an "achievement of which every doctor in America should be proud." Otto Juettner, in his book *Daniel Drake and His Followers* (1909), wrote of this episode:

> Drake was present, and, upon arising, was greeted with a demonstration [applause] such as never had been accorded to anyone on a similar occasion. The cheers and the clapping of hand were deafening and lasted for several minutes. Again and again the demonstrations started anew. Finally, when the noise subsided, Drake wanted to thank his colleagues, but his voice failed him. He seemed to be growing faint and was helped to a chair. He covered his face with his hands and wept like a child...when he gained his self-possession, [Drake said]: *"I have not lived in vain, but I wish father, mother, and Harriet [his wife] were here."*

Two years after this Daniel Drake was buried in Spring Grove Cemetery in Cincinnati next to his wife and deceased children, brother, and parents. I visit Spring Grove Cemetery with regularity—on average once a month—and more in the spring, summer, and fall to enjoy the changing scenery. I also go to learn where notable people who contributed to Cincinnati's rich past are buried. Spring Grove is a place to be reminded that generations come and go, and in that place my thoughts sometimes include an accounting of my own life and asking myself, "Am I making a difference in the lives of family, friends, and our community?"

In the cluster of the marble monuments for the Drake family, Daniel Drake's is the tallest, and with time the engraving on the marble stones have worn, making it difficult to read. Back in 1952 physicians in Cincinnati gathered to celebrate the one hundredth anniversary of Drake's death and affixed on his monument a bronze plaque making readable the original faded words:

> Sacred to the memory of Daniel Drake, a learned and distinguished physician, an able and philosophical writer, an eminent teacher of the medical art, a citizen of exemplary virtue and public spirit, a man rarely equaled in all the gentler qualities which adorn social and domestic life. His fame is indelibly written in the records of his country, his good deeds impressed on beneficent public institutions endure forever. He lived in the fear of God and died in hope of salvation. He who rests here was an early inhabitant and untiring friend of the City of Cincinnati with whose prosperity his fame is inseparably connected.

"His fame is *indelibly* written in the records of his country, his good deeds impressed on beneficent public institutions *endure forever*." In a sense, yes, this is true; few men have made the kind of mark on their field and community as Drake, the leading clinician/educator of his time in American medicine (1815–1852). Nor did his accomplishments go unnoticed by those who came after him; I first discovered Drake's name through reading a quotation in Harvey Cushing's biography of Sir William Osler (1849–1919) in which Osler observed that "everything that is good and lasted in Cincinnati could be traced back to Daniel Drake." And yet, the contributions he made have been largely lost with the passage of time. This is a fact that Juettner lamented back in 1909 when he wrote, "Posterity has done nothing for this great man. He seems to be entirely forgotten." In this generation Cincinnatians recognize the name of Drake Hospital, but do not know much, if anything, of the man. There is a subset of local historians who know of him and some of his contributions, but outside of Cincinnati he is less known and only by a small number of physicians and medical historians. The words inscribed on his monument speak to a rich, impactful multifaceted legacy and suggests that learning about his life may provide insights into why his peers said his "deeds... endure forever."

On the occasion of the University of Cincinnati's sesquicentennial celebration in 1969, Henry D. Shapiro and Zane L. Miller from UC's history department sought to honor the founder of the University of Cincinnati, Dr. Daniel Drake, by producing a volume of his writings, entitled *Physician to the West: Selected Writings of Daniel Drake on Science and Society.* Their book drew from eighteen of Drake's works on topics ranging from medical school education, notes on Cincinnati, intemperance, discipline, railroads and use of waterways, promotion of literary and social institutions, and diseases of the Ohio Valley. The book offered a brief chronology of Drake's life and the most complete bibliography of Drake's writings including 698 works published from 1804 to 1852. This book had a limited circulation and is out of print.

The impetus for this book originated with the University of Cincinnati's Bicentennial Commission and is an extension of Shapiro and Miller's work. Recognizing their book had a different intended purpose and drew on a limited number of Drake's works, members of the Bicentennial Commission considered a proposal to sample the Drake corpus more widely to give a sense of his range of activity and thought. I hope as well that this book provides an example of how a legacy can be built and can inspire readers, particularly young adults, to live a life that leads to such a legacy as Drake's.

This work reveals Drake in his own words as a person, writing about his key formative experiences, his passions, his interests in building culture in community, his use of writing to shape conversations, his thoughts on education and being an educator, and lastly his perceptions of the scope and work of a physician. His mind was active and far ranging, dedicated to learning, and intent on building and improving life for others. His valuable insights and lessons are timeless. It is my desire that his example will have an impact on readers who can appreciate the genius of the individual recognized as the founder of the University of Cincinnati and many other enduring institutions in our city.

A starting point is to ask the question what *is* a legacy? A legacy is often thought of as a monetary gift, but a legacy is about more than giving money. Each human life is a story made up of choices and actions, habits of character, experiences shared with others, responses to triumphs and failings. Life stories can range from tragic to heroic, dramatic to comedic, and through their course, communicate messages, lessons, or gifts so others may benefit. Thus, an expanded concept of legacy includes the messages we can read from a life well lived. A legacy can result from acts of offering a helping hand, using power to do good, improving and building community, educating and providing wise counsel, defining and shaping a field of endeavor, or creating technological innovations. Such lives of meaning provide lessons for their contemporaries, but in addition, examining the lives of individuals from the past can be beneficial to future generations. For any person interested in living a life of purpose and aspiring to make a difference, Daniel Drake's is an exemplary one and worthy of study. Through learning his life's lessons his legacy endures.

⊠ A Brief Introduction to Drake's Life

Daniel Drake was born in 1785 to a poor family that migrated when he was four years old from New Jersey to Mayslick, Kentucky, near the banks of the Ohio River about sixty miles upriver from Cincinnati. His formal education lasted only six months, and he spent his childhood and adolescence in the outdoors. He was the oldest of six children, and it was often his responsibility to care for his younger siblings. He took on the work of a pioneer farmer and felt the intrinsic satisfaction of doing a task well. From working alongside his father in the forest and fields and helping his mother with chores around the cabin, he learned the value and importance of being industrious. He learned to be respectful and honored his parents through his obedience. His parents saw to it that he acquired a strong moral compass, which guided his approach to others throughout his life. His parents were not well educated but valued education.

Though his formal education was limited, he learned more importantly how to teach himself. Speaking of the value of reading he said, "As to my actual attainments in learning, they were certainly quite limited, and yet I could read and examine a dictionary for the meaning of words and here is the starting point of all improvement" (1.11). He never forgot the words he learned, and he acquired an extensive vocabulary.

His early upbringing was foundational to shaping his character. Besides being self-taught, a keen observer, and industrious, he was disciplined, ambitious, and continuously sought to improve himself. But events present opportunities that call for a response and in turn, shape the person. Drake's life provides multiple examples of seizing the initiative, stepping through the open door, and making the most of opportunities he was offered.

As a young boy his father decided Drake would have a career in medicine. In 1800, aspiring doctors apprenticed themselves to an established physician. The plan for Drake to become a doctor was altered by a family tragedy. Here is a selection entitled "How Serendipity Directs Our Lives" that chronicles this time in his life:

> The long talked of project—that of "making me a doctor," had at length been finally settled in the affirmative [at age fourteen]. I was to enter on the study in a few months with my cousin, Dr. John Drake, whose education was then nearly completed, and whose genius was only equaled by his great moral purity. With this prospect before me, he was taken ill in July with typhus fever, and died in August, 1799. This was my first disappointment, and a real misfortune to me, for he would have been a good preceptor, and I could've studied at home, and thus saved father an expense which he was in no way prepared to meet.... Had Dr. John Drake lived, I should not have gone to Cincinnati to study medicine, and of a consequence never resided there. In fact, humanly speaking, my whole course of life might have been entirely different from what it has been. I should probably have become a country doctor and a member of the General assembly! His death did not turn father aside from the determination that I should study physic [medicine]. (1.15)

He was then apprenticed for four years (1800–1804) to his father's friend and the family's doctor, Dr. William Goforth, who was practicing in the young village of Cincinnati, which in 1800 had a population of 850 people. Dr. Goforth was an excellent mentor, and his partner, Dr. John Stites Jr., had trained in Philadelphia and was familiar with the writings and teachings of Dr. Benjamin Rush, the leading physician educator of his time. It was during this period as an apprentice that Drake transformed from a backwoods farmer to a full physician partner in Goforth's practice by the end of his training at age nineteen. What enabled him to achieve that remarkable transformation was the motivation not to fail and disappoint his parents, industriousness, curiosity and eagerness to learn from the standard texts and his teachers, and an amazing ability to envision the big picture of how human life is ordered and works. He was a system thinker who could see the whole while having a command of the details.

When he had finished his apprenticeship, rather than continue on with Dr. Goforth's practice, in 1805 he elected to seek further training in Philadelphia. This was a critical formative experience. Philadelphia was the leading city in the United States at the time. Greatly economizing, he attended the University of Pennsylvania and was taught by the best medical faculty in the country including Benjamin Rush, Caspar Wistar, and Benjamin Barton. It was Barton who imparted an approach to medicine that became his lifelong practice: learning by accurately describing what is seen through firsthand observation, drawing inferences from personal observations, and writing these down for the benefit of others. This is the approach of a naturalist, and in time Drake supplemented this approach by reading widely and consistently to add to his growing clinical knowledge. When he returned to Cincinnati he used this approach to prepare his first little book, *Notices on Cincinnati*, published in 1810.

It was in Philadelphia that he also saw a more refined and developed community, enriched by the arts and social institutions, and the contrast with the emerging village of Cincinnati (still under 2,500 in population) was conspicuous. After returning to Cincinnati and venturing into the surrounding region along and north of the Ohio River, he adeptly recognized the region was undeveloped, but surrounded by abundant natural resources. He saw Cincinnati's location on the Ohio River as having great potential to make it a leading city in the interior. Philadelphia was a model for what Cincinnati could be become. Drake's second book, *Statistical Notes on Cincinnati*, published in 1815, introduced Cincinnati to the rest of the United States and helped promote it as a destination city. Institutions such as government bodies, schools, banks, libraries, hospitals, museums, and societies to promote culture, all active in Philadelphia, were yet to be created. Drake wrote the following visionary statement in 1833:

> Communities, like forest, go rigid by time. They properly trained must be molded while young. Our duty, then, is quite obvious. All who have moral power, should exert it in concert. The germs of harmony must be nourished, and the roots of present contrariety or

future discord torn up and cast into the fire. Measures should be taken to mold a uniform system of manners and customs, out of the diversified elements which are scattered over the west.... The whole should successively lend a helping hand to all the parts, on the great subject of education from the primary school to the university.... In short, we should foster Western genius, encourage Western writers, patronize Western publishers, augment the number of Western readers, and create a Western heart. (2.11)

It was in Philadelphia that the seeds were sown for an academic medical career, which germinated during his first decade of clinical practice. By 1815 the idea of becoming a teacher of medicine became a prime ambition. To teach he would need to have more training and an MD degree, and he once again returned in that year to Philadelphia to the University of Pennsylvania to acquire that degree.

He had learned what made an effective teacher and was an eloquent and inspiring lecturer who frequently used questions and practical examples to engage the learner. He also saw the deficiencies in the current state of medical education and in the knowledge and skills of the average medical practitioner. Medicine needed higher standards for training and practice, and during his academic career he led efforts to reform medical education. It was his zeal for high standards, both for himself and his colleagues, that contributed to friction when he first started the Medical College of Ohio in 1819. Two years later his colleagues, full of envy and jealousy, voted him out of the very school he started. Undeterred from this early failure to lead, he retained a lifelong commitment to improving medical education accompanied by high standards of conduct and character.

His essays on medical education, first presented as journal articles, were later published as a collection in 1832 in a classic volume, *Practical Essays on Medical Education in the Medical Profession in the United States.* His thoughts on medical education were innovative and far ahead of his time, defining the stages of a medical education, setting high standards for prerequisites and selection of medical students, lengthening the course of medical education, teaching clinical medicine at the bedside in teaching hospitals, having medical schools under local control but accountable to the state governments, and advising on how to learn in practice. Fielding H. Garrison in his book *History of Medicine* (1929) said, "His celebrated essays on Medical Education,...are, far and away, the most important contribution ever made to the subject in this country. They are written in a style which, for clarity and beauty is, even today, a perfect model of what such writing should be."

⊠ HIS WRITINGS AS A LENS TO DISCOVER HIS LEGACY

Daniel Drake was a prolific writer leaving a corpus of seven books and over 700 journal articles, letters, and spoken addresses. These works provide insights into his legacy, the gifts he created and left for posterity, and they provide a guide for anyone wishing to lead a life of meaning and purpose for the benefit of others.

His love for reading was the basis for becoming an excellent writer. He followed Benjamin Franklin's rules for improving his writing and added a few of his own. Commonplace books, journals, and letters were early outlets, followed by scientific reports and then his small book, *Statistical Notes on Cincinnati*. His update and expansion of this book in 1815 established his reputation nationally. Early in his career he founded a debating society where papers were prepared and given by the members, and later he was asked to give addresses to many conferences and meetings. He wrote poetry and did so for those closest to him or for special occasions. After practicing for twenty years and teaching medicine for twelve, he became the editor of the *Western Journal of the Medical and Physical Sciences* and its successor the *Western Journal of Medicine and Surgery* from 1827 to 1850. This role required regular editorials and opportunities for original articles, brief news reports, book reviews, and obituaries. He was able to write with sarcasm in response to quackery or strong biting polemic when attacked publicly. His book on cholera, drawing from international sources, was published four months before the cholera epidemic of 1832 entered the United States, and is an example of his public service by providing a timely and comprehensive summary of what was then known. He was also a meticulous historian, leaving a memoir of the early beginnings of the "Miami Country" (the region around and including Cincinnati) and a history of early physicians in Cincinnati. As mentioned earlier he published his classic essays on medical education, *Practical Essays on Medical Education in the Medical Profession in the United States*, as a collection in 1832.

I discovered Drake's writings when I came to the University of Cincinnati for residency training and became acquainted with the Cincinnati Medical Heritage Center on the Medical Campus. Here I developed a relationship with Billie Broaddus who was the curator at the time, and my fascination with Drake began when she introduced me to the center's Drake Collection of primary materials. She gave me a little book the center produced in 1985: *Daniel Drake MD, Frontiersman of the Mind*. This was a collection put together by Dr. Charles Aring that included addresses to medical students that had never been published before, and one in particular stood out, entitled "The Formation of Professional Character" given in 1835 at the start of first session of the second Cincinnati medical school Drake started, the Medical Department of the Cincinnati College. In this address Drake outlines the character qualities needed to be successful as a physician, and I saw similarities in thought and style between William Osler and Drake and began to wonder how Drake potentially influenced Osler, who taught and practiced a generation later.

Drake's ability to see, understand, and transpose that understanding into descriptive prose was evident from that first essay. He could adopt his style to the audience—so his letters to his children are very conversational, his contribution to legislation was to the point, his books were exhaustive and comprehensive, his editorials could be informational or satirical, his clinical case descriptions were concise yet detailed, his speeches were laced with visual images, his lectures included engaging questions, and so on. He thought through problems of his day with a freshness, thoroughness, and originality while highlighting enduring principles relevant for any time period. From my medical school days I have gravitated to physician writers who have addressed the importance of character, and few have spoken to the question of character and legacy in their lives and deeds more than Daniel Drake.

And yet, for all the wisdom and foresight of his educational essays (and I have incorporated selections from Drake's writings into lectures and classes), a review of his vast corpus identified the practical lessons collected in this book, to answer the central questions: "What was Drake's legacy?" and "How was it achieved?" Consider this selection, entitled "Responsibility Grows Us":

> In the midst of this last effort, however, a family afflic-
> tion arose, which greatly interrupted my studies. Father
> got a severe injury on his foot, which partially mortified,
> and three or four of the children were taken down with
> the ague [malaria] and fever—the first time that that
> disease had ever visited us. In my letter two years ago,
> I must have mentioned these facts, but probably did not
> tell you (boastingly) that when the care of everything
> turned on mother and myself, my heart grew big with

the emotions which such calamities naturally inspire, and with the feeling of responsibility that was quite as natural, producing in my actions their proper fruit; and father and mother commended me for my labors, both indoors and out. To speak of the whole matter frankly, I look back, even from this distant point of time, 47 years, to my conduct with approbation and pleasure. What a precious reward (referring to this life only) there is and striving to do what trying occasions require of us! (1.16)

A person could read this as an interesting letter to his children for understanding Drake's thought and life, but reading with intention to identify a life lesson (the method used here) takes it beyond a casual understanding. When the reader enters into feelings and thoughts the story arouses, one can identify, in one's own life, random events that called for an opportunity to assume responsibility or not. Do we seek to understand these common life experiences and how we responded to them? Or do we let them pass by, missing their deeper meaning?

ORGANIZATION AND APPROACH OF THE BOOK

The selections from Drake's writings are organized thematically, grouped in terms of the five dimensions of human experience captured on the bronze plaque on his monument by his peers and contemporaries: as a man, a citizen, a writer, a teacher, and a physician. I sought selections from his writings that would relate to or fit into one of these five categories. Admittedly there is overlap—that is, one selection could potentially be included in another section. But I found it a useful scheme to organize the selections and lessons. As I read through Drake's writings I purposely avoided material where his thoughts were clearly dated or failed to illustrate a lesson about legacy building, and thus, what is included here is an incomplete picture of Drake's thoughts. A critical biography would be necessary to properly present all the rich complexities of Drake's life and thought, and that was not the purpose of this book.

Some guiding questions for populating the selections into these sections included:

Man: What was his character? What were his formative experiences? How did he choose his career?

Citizen: What institutions did he build? From what sources did he get his vision? How did he build institutions? What role did partnerships play?

Writer: How did he learn to write? What outlets did he use to write? Why did he write? What are representative examples of his different writing styles?

Educator: What was his approach to teaching? What practical pedagogy did he adopt? Why was he considered a master educator? What principles for reform of education did he offer? How did he think physicians should be educated?

Physician: How did he conceive the role and scope of a physician? What were his insights on the physician's relationship to the patient and offering care and hope to patients when very little could be done? How did he describe the stages of becoming a master physician? How did he view the causes of disease? How did he approach treatment in that era when so little was available? Why was he considered a great physician?

The title of each selection identifies important life lessons. Consider as an example "How Serendipity Directs Our Lives" from above. First, life's random events are opportunities to develop an appreciation of serendipity. Second, taking on the mantle of responsibility rather than observing others is a means to growing our skills and knowledge. We must seek out tasks, volunteer for them as a means of lifelong learning and growing new capacities.

It is my hope that readers will engage this book with questions in mind about living a life that leads to a positive legacy. What did Drake achieve with his life? How did he do it? What were his formative experiences? What were the means he used? What are the life lessons that are presented in each section that are relevant to me? What can I do to develop my gifts and talents further? Using some of these lessons, where can I make a positive impact in my circle of influence? To assist the reader with personalizing the life lessons, each selection includes questions for reflection designed to engage the reader about the theme raised by the selection. It is a way to model how to read with questions in mind. The reflection questions are a way of teaching, too. I hope they will prompt the reader to personalize the theme of the selection in some useful way.

Daniel Drake, through his multiple roles as man, citizen, writer, educator, and physician, created an enduring legacy—through participating as a citizen concerned with improving his community, through his role as a gifted writer to inform and shape the conversation in public and professional circles, through his role as an educator inspiring learners and setting high expectations and standards, and through his role as a clinician who saw the big picture and as caregiver who took a broad, systematic approach to understanding the patient and community in a time when the practice of medicine was yet to be founded on a firm scientific foundation.

These were Drake's gifts. There is much to learn from this very articulate and passionate individual who saw his community transformed in his lifetime from a small village into the sixth largest city in the United States. He was a major catalyst and contributor to that transformation. It has been said he did much to promote the intellectual life of Cincinnati. His approach to living a life of purpose and meaning is not limited to him, or his time, but serves as an example to anyone who also wishes to leave an enduring legacy—becoming a person of great character, addressing the current needs of the community, helping grow and improve the culture, finding ways to communicate to others the lessons learned, and working to become a master in one's chosen field.

Those lessons remain relevant and needed today, particularly when individuals have an abundance of offerings to occupy their time. One of the most pressing challenges for those living today is to develop one's sense of purpose. Many wish to live a life that makes a difference. There is a level of pressure young people put on themselves to achieve and perform. Accompanying that is a high level of impatience, to do it now, and in turn, failing to recognize that a meaning-filled life takes time to unfold. I briefly mentioned the value of recognizing formative experiences. Drake's life is an exemplary model; his various means and methods of engaging his community as a citizen, a writer, an educator, and a physician map out an approach that can be followed by anyone.

It is my hope that the selections contained in this book, and the questions with each selection, will make Daniel Drake's work and life accessible to a new generation who will find practical life lessons and be aided in their quest to create their own legacies, as Drake did, through "good deeds" that will "endure forever."

⬛ A NOTE ON TEXT

At the end of the book is a more detailed chronology of Drake's life and a bibliography of the writings cited in this book. The main corpus of the book is divided into five sections, one for each area of Drake's legacy: Man, Citizen, Writer, Educator, and Physician. Selections from primary sources were chosen to highlight a specific theme pertinent to that section. The selections are in Drake's own words with moderate correction or modernization of spelling and punctuation. In some instances, paragraphs from a larger selection were edited and arranged to present the main points in fewer words. The selections are introduced with a title that serves as an aid to identify a specific lesson. Each selection is followed by a set of questions or comments "for reflection" to assist the reader in personalizing the selection or for using in group discussions with goal of applying the lesson. Good fortune from your reading and reflecting.

—Philip M. Diller, MD, PhD

Senior Associate Dean of Educational Affairs; Professor, Department of Family and Community Medicine; and Chair, Advisory Board, Henry R. Winkler Center for the History of the Health Professions, College of Medicine, University of Cincinnati

LEAVING A LEGACY

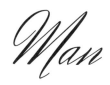

Man

*"A man rarely equaled in all the gentler qualities
which adorn social and domestic life"*

"Return to the primitive settlement, and meditate on the circumstances under
which I passed what, I suppose, in reference to the formation of character, to
have been the most important period of my life—that in which it got its set."
—*Daniel Drake, January 14, 1848*

1.1 *Social Lessons Growing Up*

1.2 *Lessons from Your Family of Origin*

1.3 *Parental Examples as Strong Shapers of Behavior*

1.4 *Inheriting Your Temperament and Receiving the Counsel of Your Parents*

1.5 *Develop the Habit of Ordering the First Part of the Day*

1.6 *Learn to Execute a Task Faithfully*

1.7 *Take Pleasure in Hard Work and Learn to Be Patient to See a Desired Outcome*

1.8 *Train for Duty and Obedience*

1.9 *Use All Your Senses to Learn*

1.10 *Develop Your Imagination and Curiosity by Regularly Playing Outdoors*

1.11 *The Books That Shape Us*

1.12 *Acquire the Fundamentals of Learning*

1.13 *Learn to Defend Yourself*

1.14 *Recognize Personal Deficiencies and Work to Eliminate Them*

1.15 *How Serendipity Directs Our Lives*

1.16 *Responsibility Grows Us*

1.17 *Learn Deeply Instead of Superficially*

1.18   *Acquire a Worldview*

1.19   *Learn from Your First Illness Experience*

1.20   *Deciding on Your Career*

1.21   *Parental Expectations and Sacrifices*

1.22   *Beginning My Medical Apprenticeship*

1.23   *Lessons from a Mentor*

1.24   *Become Self-Aware and Learn to Appreciate What Motivates You to Achieve*

1.25   *Seek to Develop Your Intellect and Character*

1.26   *Cultivate Punctuality and Patience*

1.27   *Train Deliberately for Character*

1.28   *Be Industrious—Build Your Capacity for Work*

1.29   *The Benefits of Industriousness*

1.30   *Learn to Be Methodical to Maximize Your Productiveness*

1.31   *Cultivate a Meekness of Spirit to Counter Human Pride and Hubris*

1.32   *The Value of an Observation Road Trip in Your Formative Years*

1.33   *Useful Knowledge as the Basis of Societal Happiness*

1.34   *Enjoy a Spouse as Friend, Co-laborer, and Motivator*

1.35   *Contrasting Legacies*

1.36   *Do Not Rest on the Accomplishments of Your Ancestors*

Chapter One

— *Drake's early childhood fascination with nature and the outdoors helped motivate a later interest in medicine and science as a teenager and adult.*

— *Drake married his wife Harriet Sisson in 1807 and went on to have five children, three of whom lived into adulthood. His wife died at age 39, and he never married again. Drake was a devoted husband, father, and grandfather who prioritized spending time with his family and grandchildren.*

— *An avid traveler, Drake visited over a dozen states in his life, often taking long trips to explore wide areas of the country at a time.*

— *He spent his childhood in Kentucky, his teenage years in Cincinnati, and went to medical school in Pennsylvania. He spent his adult life between Kentucky and Ohio as a father and physician.*

▨ AUTHOR INTRODUCTION

What prepares a person for a life that makes a positive difference in the world? A person who understands the times in which he lives and recognizes the needs in a community has the seeds to grow a legacy. But more than knowing the times or recognizing needs, a person must have initiative, industry, and the ability to influence. A person's character and capacities take shape in the formative period of life: guidance by parents, teachers, and mentors, developing a curiosity about life, experiencing increased responsibility, and growing the ability to learn as you live.

The selections in this section from Daniel Drake's writings provide insight into his formative influences that started him on his path as a learner, created his philosophy of life and understanding of the human experience, and developed his character traits that included ambition, initiative, discipline, industriousness, commitment to excellence, and a heightened sense of duty and service. These traits are common to individuals who leave a legacy.

✖ 1.1 Social Lessons Growing Up

Mayslick, although scarcely a village, was at once an emporium and capital for a tract of country 6 or 8 miles in diameter, and embracing several hundred families, of which those in father's neighborhood were tolerably fair specimens.... Mayslick was a colony of East Jersey people, amounting to an aggregate of 52 souls...thirteen families, and I think there were more. The immigrants from the other states were almost entirely Virginians and Marylanders. All were country people by birth and residence; all were illiterate in various degrees; and all were poor or in moderate circumstances; a majority or, at least, a moiety were small freeholders.... The mechanic arts practiced at that time were only those which are inseparable with civilization. The blacksmith, house carpenter, turner, tanner, shoemaker, tailor, weaver, and such like, made the whole, and all were very commonplace in skill. The great occupation was clearing off the forest and cultivating the rich and fresh new soil....

Uncle Abraham Drake kept a store, and Shotwell and Morris kept taverns; beside them were a few poor mechanics. Uncle Cornelius Drake was a farmer.... With this limited population, it seems, even down to this time, wonderful to me that such gatherings and such scenes should have been transacted there....

The infant capital was the local seat of justice; and Saturday was for many years, at all times, I might say, the regular term time. Instead of trying cases at home, two or three justices of the peace would come to the "Lick" on that day, and hold their separate courts. This, of course, brought thither all the litigants of the neighborhood, with their friends and witnesses; all who wished to purchase at the store would postpone their visit to the same day; all who had to replenish their jugs of whiskey did the same thing; all who had business with others expect- ed to meet them there, as our city merchants, at noon, expected to meet each other on "change"; finally, all who thirsted after drink, fun, frolic, or fighting, of course were present. Thus, Saturday was a day largely suspended of field labor, but devoted to public business, social pleasure, dissipation, and beastly drunkenness. You might suppose the presence of civil magistrates would have repressed some of the vices, but it was not so. Each day provided a bill of fare for the next. A new trade in horses, another horse race, a cock-fight, or a dog-fight, a wrestling match, or a pitched battle between two bullies, who in fierce encounter would lie on the ground scratching, pulling hair, choking, gouging out each other's eyes, and biting off each other's noses, in the manner of bulldogs, while a Roman circle of interested lookers-on would encourage the respective gladiators with shouts which a passing demon might have mistaken for those of hell....

I need scarcely tell you that these scenes did not contaminate me. They were quite too gross and wicked to be attractive. On the other hand they excited disgust and received from father the strongest condemnation.... My mother still more perhaps than my father...protected me.

> *Blest is the heedless little boy*
> *To whom is given,*
> *(The boon of heaven)*
> *A pious mother, ever kind.*
> *Yet never to his wand'rings blind:*
> *Who watches every erring step*
> *In holy fear,*
> *And drops a tear*
> *Of pity on the chast'ning rod*
> *Then strikes, and points, in prayer to God.*

Pioneer Life in Kentucky: A Series of Reminiscential Letters from Daniel Drake, M.D., of Cincinnati to His Children. Edited by Charles D. Drake. Cincinnati: Robert Clark & Co., 1870. 180, 183–185, 187–190.

READER REFLECTION

1. *Growing up who were the people who made up your community? Ethnicity? Level of education? Occupations? Values? How did this shape you?*
2. *Was there a rhythm of social events through the seasons? Were there social events from which your parents protected you?*
3. *Who were the adults in your community who guided your early development, and how did they do so?*

✸ 1.2 LESSONS FROM YOUR FAMILY OF ORIGIN

When I was twelve years old, sister Lizzy was ten, and father and mother began to find assistance from us at the same time. Still, up to my departure from home to study medicine, my old functions were performed, more or less, on rainy days and Sundays, on wash days, and every night and morning. My pride was in the labors of the field, but taste and duty held me, as occasion required, to the duties of the house. The time has been (perhaps should be still), when I looked back upon the years thus spent, as lost. Lost as it respects my destiny in life; lost as to distinction in my profession; lost as to influence in the generation to which I belong. But might I have not been rocked in the cradle of affluence, been surrounded by servants and tutors, exempt from every kind of labor, and indulged in every lawful gratification, and yes have at last fallen short of the limited and humble respectability which I now enjoy? In the half century which has elapsed since I began to emerge from those duties, I have certainly seen many who, enjoying all that I have named, still came to naught, were blighted, and if they did not fall from the parent bough, could not sustain themselves after the natural separation, but perished when they were expected to rise in strength and beauty. Who can tell that such might not have been my fate? The truth is, that I was the whole time in a school (I will not any longer say, of adversity, but) of probation and discipline, and was only deprived of the opportunities afforded by the school of letters. Great and precious as these are to him who is afterward to cultivate literature and science, they are not the whole. They impart a certain kind of knowledge, and strengthen the memory, but they leave many important principles of our nature undeveloped, and therefore cannot guarantee future usefulness or fame.

I was preserved from many temptations, and practically taught self-denial, because indulgence beyond certain narrow limits was so much out of the question as not to be thought of. I was taught to practice economy, and to think of money as a thing not to be expended on luxuries, but to be used for useful ends. I was taught the value of learning, by being denied the opportunities for acquiring more than a pittance. I was taught the value of time, by having more to do day after day than could be well accomplished. I was molded to do many things, if not absolutely at the same time, in such quick succession as almost to render them identical; a habit which I have found of great advantage to me through life. But better than all these, I grew up with love and obedience to my mother, and received from her an early moral training, to which, in conjunction with that of my father, I owe, perhaps, more of my humble success in life, and of my humble preparation for the life to come, than to any other influence. She was still more illiterate than my father, but was pious, and could read the Bible, *Rippon's Hymns*, and *Pilgrim's Progress*. Her natural understanding was tolerable only, but she comprehended the principles of domestic and Christian duty, and sought to inculcate them. This she never did by protracted lectures, but mixed them up with all our daily labors. Thus, my mother was always by my side, and ready with her reproof, or admonition, or rewarding smile, as occasion required or opportunity arose.... Her theory of morals was abundantly simple—*God has said it!* The Bible forbids this, and commands that, and God will punish you if you act contrary to his word! What philosopher could have risen so high? How simple and yet how sublime!

Pioneer Life in Kentucky: A Series of Reminiscential Letters from Daniel Drake, M.D., of Cincinnati to His Children. Edited by Charles D. Drake. Cincinnati: Robert Clark & Co., 1870. 109–111.

Reader Reflection

1. *Attending a "School of Letters" and growing up in affluence does not guarantee success. What important "principles of our nature" (character) also need to be developed that increase our likelihood of success?*
2. *Drake maximized learning while living. Consider how that is done.*

1.3 Parental Examples as Strong Shapers of Behavior

It has been said, that most great men have had talented mothers. How much of their superiority might have been a birth-right, we need not stop to inquire, but, there is little doubt, that much of it, as far as the mother was concerned, arose from her instruction and discipline—training the faculties and affections by times, insisting on their supremacy over the appetites, and directing even the tottering steps of infancy into paths, that finally, led up to the temple of fame; a height that is never reached by those who loiter on the way to eat and drink beyond the comforts of nature, or join in the wild revelries, or prosecute the schemes of vanity, avarice, or revenge....

The first great affection developed [in human life] is the love of the mother; to which succeeds, in due time, that for the father, and at length, (the conduct and character of both parents being alike), the affection for both seems, in general, to be equal. Now, at the earliest dawn of intellect, the child be rewarded and punished through this affection. When the mother frowns upon it or turns away her face, the sun of its happiness is dimmed—it is distressed and punished, through the medium of its filial affection. On the other hand, when the soft music of her voice falls upon its ear, and her countenance beams with love and praise, it rejoices as the chilled and tender lily of spring expands, when the clouds are chased away, and the fountains of light and heat are opened afresh.

Here then is the first, and, let me add, the greatest of the means of moral government, which God has given us; and no mother honors the name, or deserves to be blessed with children, who neglects its use. Early and skillfully exercised, it fixes over the child a dominion, that, like the permanent colors which the light of the sun stamps upon the opening rose, must be felt, till the individual is gathered with that mother in the grave. To *maintain* the influence, the parents, however, must attend to all that is necessary. They should view the child as having a rational soul, capable, as it grows in years, of observing and reasoning, and having other desires and wants, than those which, through infancy, make it cleave to its mother's bosom as the source of all its enjoyments, and its place of refuge in every danger. They should know, that to preserve an influence founded on filial affection, they must, as the child increases in age and knowledge, keep themselves in its respect and veneration. To do this, they should administer the reward of their approbation, and inflict the punishment of their displeasure on such occasions only as demand them, and apportion them to the acts that are to be rewarded or punished. They must, in the very midst of their chastisements, convince the child of their affection, and that they are but discharging a duty of love. They should again and again recite the law of duty it has violated, and instruct it anew as far as practicable, on the reasons for the law; thus, making it conscious that the punishment was merited, and will, finally, be for its own happiness. In this way, they will associate mental instruction with mental pain, and, at the same time, appear as benefactors instead of tyrants. They will excite repentance, which never comes from punishment unaccompanied with the conviction of error, and instead of anger inspire a sentiment of reverence, when parental government is placed on a foundation that cannot be shaken.

To accomplish this great object, however, it is indispensable that parents should look to their own conduct. In their lives they must evince, that they are governed by moral laws, which are but a stretching out to greater objects and duties, of the laws they lay down for the government of the child. They should come into the family tribunal with clean hands, and engrave on the rod of correction, *"Let him that is without sin, cast the first stone."*

How is it possible that parents who give themselves up to passion and caprice, to deception and petty falsehoods, to instability of principle and fickleness of pursuit, to backbitings, to gluttony and drunkenness, to profanity, grossness, and impiety, can by any rewards or punishments, make themselves objects of veneration, or acquire over their offspring a moral power? To do this, they must practice what they enjoin, show obedience to the laws of society and God, and present themselves as examples of whatever purity human nature can acquire.

"Discipline: Discourse on the Philosophy of Family, School, and College Discipline." *Transactions of the Fourth Annual Meeting of the Western Literary Institute and College of Professional Teachers.* Cincinnati: Josiah Drake Publisher, 1835. 45–47.

READER REFLECTION

1. *What was the motivation for discipline given to you by your parents? Did they give reasons why they were disciplining you?*
2. *What were the most valuable lessons you received from your parents?*

✠ 1.4 INHERITING YOUR TEMPERAMENT AND RECEIVING THE COUNSEL OF YOUR PARENTS

While occupying the first cabin, my mother one day made a call at a neighboring cabin, where a woman was churning. Tired out with diet of bread and meat, mother fixed her heart on a drink of buttermilk, but said nothing. When the butter was ladled out and the churn set aside, with the delicious beverage, for which she was too proud to ask (and which the other perhaps did not think of giving) she hastily left the house and took a good crying spell. Thus you see whence came my propensity, and Dove's and Charlie's [his children], for crying. We all, in fact, resemble my mother in temperament, of which this is one of the proofs; while another is our hereditary propensity is to go to sleep in church! Your brother Charles and yourself [Echo] have the temperament of your mother and my father.

...This original principle of my nature [cautiousness], which throughout life has given me some trouble and saved me from some, was, perhaps, augmented by two causes: 1st. For a good while I had no male companions. The sons of my uncles were too old to play with me, and I did not associate much with those near my own age in the families of Morris and Shotwell, as my parents did not wish it, and they lived further off than my uncles. My cousin Osee Drake, uncle Abraham's oldest daughter, and cousin Polly Drake, uncle Cornelius's daughter, both a little older than I, were for four or five years my chief companions. We agreed well, for they were good children; and while they contributed to soften my manners, and quicken my taste for female companionship, they no doubt increased my timidity.

2nd. My mother was, by nature and religious education, a non-combatant, and throughout the whole period of her tutelage, that is, till I went from home to study medicine, sought to impress upon me not to fight. Father had, constitutionally, a great amount of caution, but was personally brave, and, as I now recollect, did not concur with the counsels of mother.

Pioneer Life in Kentucky: A Series of Reminiscential Letters from Daniel Drake, M.D., of Cincinnati to His Children. Edited by Charles D. Drake. Cincinnati: Robert Clark & Co., 1870. 10–11.

READER REFLECTION

1. *Are you an emotional person who easily cries or just the opposite? Did you "inherit" this from your parents?*
2. *What traits do you think you have inherited from your father? Your mother?*

✠ 1.5 DEVELOP THE HABIT OF ORDERING THE FIRST PART OF THE DAY

Father and mother were early risers, and I was drilled into the same habit before I was 10 years old. In winter we were generally up before the dawn of day. After making a fire, the first thing was feeding and foddering the horses, hogs, sheep, and cattle. Corn, husks, blades, and tops had to be distributed, and times without number I have done this by the light of the moon reflected on the snow. This done at an earlier hour than common, old Lion [his dog] and I sometimes took a little hunt in the woods; but were never very successful. I had a taste for hunting, but neither time nor genius for any great achievement in that way. Among the pleasant recollections of those mornings are the red-birds, robins, and snow-birds, which made their appearance to pick up the scattering grains of corn where the cattle had been fed.

Pioneer Life in Kentucky: A Series of Reminiscential Letters from Daniel Drake, M.D., of Cincinnati to His Children. Edited by Charles D. Drake. Cincinnati: Robert Clark & Co., 1870. 76–77.

READER REFLECTION

1. *Do you have routine habits to start the day? What are they? Could they be improved?*
2. *How important is the start to the day to you?*

✥ 1.6 Learn to Execute a Task Faithfully

I remember another calamitous event of those days. When about six years old, I was sent to borrow a little salt of one of the neighbors. Salt at that time was worth about three dollars a bushel, or twelve times [the cost] at present. It was a small quantity, tied up in paper, and when I had gotten about half way home, the paper tore, and most of the precious grains rolled out on the ground. As I write, the anguish I felt at the sight seems almost to be revived. I had not then learned that the spilling of salt is portentous, but felt that it was a great present affliction, and apprehended that I should be blamed or scolded. Mother had, moreover, *taught me* to consider the waste of bread, or anything that was scarce and could be used as food, as sinful. In this instance she thought, I believe, that the paper had not been properly tied. When I recur to this and other incidents, which I cannot definitely relate, *I discover that it was an original trait of character with me, to aim at faithful execution of whatever was confided to me, and to feel unhappy if, through neglect or misfortune, I made a failure.* To this hour, I am more solicitous about that which is instructed to me than that which is entirely my own; and hence I have given a great deal of time to public affairs, on a small scale to be sure, but often at the expense of my private interests.

Pioneer Life in Kentucky: A Series of Reminiscential Letters from Daniel Drake, M.D., of Cincinnati to His Children. Edited by Charles D. Drake. Cincinnati: Robert Clark & Co., 1870. 29.

Reader Reflection
1. *How do you view and approach the tasks that others give you to do? How do you feel when you fail to execute them properly?*
2. *Do you strive to do tasks well and to the best of your ability?*

✥ 1.7 Take Pleasure in Hard Work and
Learn to Be Patient to See a Desired Outcome

The summer of 1794, when I was in my ninth year,...was a new era. The land father acquired was covered with an unbroken forest, which must be cleared away, and a new cabin erected. Father was still too poor to hire a laborer for steady work, and was himself far from being a robust and vigorous man. My health was good and my spirit willing; I might, therefore, render some assistance to this new enterprise; and accordingly master Curry's hickory [his schoolmaster] and myself parted, never to meet again. I was provided with a small axe; father had a larger, and a mattock for grubbing. Thus equipped, with some bread and meat wrapped in a towel, we charged upon the beautiful blue ash and buckeye grove, in the midst of which he proposed to erect his cabin. Many days, however, did not pass before each received a wound! Of the two, father's was the most honorable. Getting his mattock fast under the roots of a grub, and making an effort to disengage it, in which he stooped too far forward, it suddenly came out, and he brought, by a jerk, the axe extremity of the implement against his forehead, making a gash through to the bone. Mine, which did not happen on the same day, was made by a jack-knife, which passed more rapidly through a crust of bread than I expected, and made a deep wound across the ball of my left hand, the scar from which remained till it was obliterated by my great burn, thirty-four years afterward. The loss of blood was not sufficient in either case to arrest the march of improvement, and, day by day, we made new conquests over all that stood in our way. Shrubs and bushes were grubbed up; trees under a foot were cut down, and those of a larger diameter "girdled," except such as would make good logs for the projected cabin, or could be easily mauled into rails. It was father's business, of course, to do the heavy chopping; mine, to hack down the saplings, and cut off the limbs of trees and pile them into brush heaps.

The brush was of course burnt up as fast as it was cut, and of all the labor in the forest, I consider that of dragging and burning the limbs of the trees the most delightful. To me it made toil a pleasure. The rapid disappearance of what was thrown upon the fire gave the feeling of progress; the flame was cheering; the crackling sound imparted animation; the columns of smoke wound their way upward, in graceful curves, among the tall green trees left standing; and the limbs of the twigs of the hickory sent forth a balmy and aromatic odor....

...Among the labors of the latter three years of my country life (age 12–15), was that of mauling rails. This was generally done in winter, and although a most laborious work, I took delight in it, and still recollect it with pleasure. A green blue-ash was my choice, for it was easy to chop and easy to split; but I often had to encounter a dead honey-locust in the field, which was a very different affair. When I was fourteen I could cut and split seventy-five rails a day out of the former, and from forty to fifty out of the latter. Still I was not large for my age, but was inured with labor, and (why I cannot explain) was willing to pursue it either alone or with father. When I got a tough log the wedges and "gluts" would fly out on being struck a hard blow. Gentle taps were necessary to get them well entered. I have often observed since, that many failures occur in the enterprises of human life from want of patience in giving the gentle taps which are necessary in beginning them.

Pioneer Life in Kentucky: A Series of Reminiscential Letters from Daniel Drake, M.D., of Cincinnati to His Children. Edited by Charles D. Drake. Cincinnati: Robert Clark & Co., 1870. 34–36, 70.

Reader Reflection

1. *Do you find pleasure in your work? Who in your life is responsible for this?*
2. *Have you learned that work done incrementally "in small taps" will in time accomplish a difficult task rather than putting it off and rushing to get it done under a time pressure?*

1.8 Train for Duty and Obedience

Up to the time of my leaving home, at the age of fifteen, my mother never had a "hired girl," except in sickness; and father never purchased a slave, for two substantial reasons: first, he had not the means; and second, he was opposed to slavery that he would not have accepted the best negro in Kentucky as a gift, provided he would have been compelled to keep him as a slave. Now and then he hired one, male or female, by the day, from some neighboring master (white hirelings being scarce), but he or mother never failed to give the slave something in return for the service. In this destitution of domestic help, and with from three to six children, of which I was the oldest, you will readily perceive that she had urgent need, daily and nightly, of all the assistance I could give her. To this service, I suppose, I was naturally well adapted, for I do not now recollect that it was ever repugnant to my feelings. At all events I acquiesced in it as a matter of duty—a thing of course; for what could she do, how get on, without my aid? I do not think, however, that I reasoned upon it like a moralist, but merely followed the promptings of those filial instincts of obedience, duty, and co-operation which are among the elements of a system of moral philosophy.

Pioneer Life in Kentucky: A Series of Reminiscential Letters from Daniel Drake, M.D., of Cincinnati to His Children. Edited by Charles D. Drake. Cincinnati: Robert Clark & Co., 1870. 90–91.

Reader Reflection

1. *Do you suppose Drake helped his mother out of feelings of love?*

2. *How does seeing work as a duty influence how a person performs the work?*
3. *What is the outcome if a person has no sense of duty?*

◩ 1.9 Use All Your Senses to Learn

The distant water-mill of which I have spoken, was two mile above the Blue Licks. It was famous for its salt. Eight hundred gallons of water had to be boiled down to obtain a bushel! Father's mode of paying for it was by taking corn or hay; for the region round about it produced neither. It was my privilege first to accompany him when I was about eleven years old. By that time he had got a small meadow. He took as much hay as two horses could draw, and after traversing a rugged and hilly road, bartered it for a bushel of salt. The trip was instructive and deeply interesting. I again passed through a zone of oak wood, and when three miles from the springs, we came to an open country, and the surface of which presented nothing but moss-covered rocks interspersed with red cedars. Not a single house or any work of art broke the solemn grandeur of the scene, and the impression it made was indelible. I here first observed the connection between rocks and evergreens, and have never seen it since without recurring to this first and wildest sight—even now a bright vision of the mind. Thus I had seen three varieties of the earth's surface, and three modifications of its natural productions. I had tasted the salt water, seen the rude evaporating furnaces, and smelt the salt and sulphurous vapor which arose in columns from them. I had learned that the immense herds of buffalo had, before the settlement of the country, frequented the spot, destroyed the shrubs and herbage around, trodden up the ground, and prepared it for being washed away by the rain, until the rocks were left bare; finally, I was told that around the licks, sunk in the mud, there had been found the bones of animals much larger than buffalo or any other then known in the country. Thus my knowledge of zoology was extended, and I received a first lesson in geology. I knew more than I had done, and could tell my mother and sisters of strange sights which they had never seen. Those sights, and other which I now and then saw, gave, I believe, a decided impulse to the love of nature implanted in the heart of every child, and to them I ascribe, in part, that taste, which, at the age of sixty, rendered my travels for professional inquiry into new regions of the diversified and boundless West, a feast at which I never cloyed. Had I at that time been incarcerated within the walls of an academy conjugating Latin verbs, or learning the Greek alpha-betas, I might possibly have become a man of erudition, but have lost, perhaps, that love of nature, which has been to me throughout life an exhaustless source of enjoyment. This, at least, is a harmless, perhaps even a praiseworthy speculation, for it is certainly commendable to submit gracefully to our deprivations, and sophistry cannot be condemned when employed to reconcile us to the conditions that are irremediable.

Pioneer Life in Kentucky: A Series of Reminiscential Letters from Daniel Drake, M.D., of Cincinnati to His Children. Edited by Charles D. Drake. Cincinnati: Robert Clark & Co., 1870. 61–62.

READER REFLECTION

1. *When did you first become aware of using all your senses to be "fully present" at a place or event?*
2. *How well do you try to use all your senses to experience what is around you?*
3. *How well do you translate such "total sensory" information into understanding?*

1.10 DEVELOP YOUR IMAGINATION AND CURIOSITY BY REGULARLY PLAYING OUTDOORS

If I were to write a recipe for making great and good men and women, I would direct the family to be placed in the woods, reared on simple food, dressed in plain clothes, made to participate in rural and domestic enjoyment, allowed to range through the groves and tickets, but required a part of every day to give themselves up to the instruction of competent and accomplished teachers, until they were 14 or 16 years of age. In my case the last element was wanting; and, therefore, you must not judge of my system by myself.

The very loneliness of our situation led me to seek for new society and amusement in the woods, as often as opportunity offered. But they were in themselves attractive. To my young mind there was in them a kind of mystery. *They excited my imagination. They awakened my curiosity.* They were exhaustless in variety. There was always something ahead. Some new or queer object might be expected, and thus anticipation was sustained. To go from the family fireside, from the midst of large and little babies, and cats and kittens, into the woods for society, may seem to you rather paradoxical, but it was not so in fact. Familiar objects lost their wonted effect, and we may become solitary in their midst.

But, to find men in trees, and women in bushes, and children in the flowers, and to be refreshed by them, one must be a little imaginative, and so I was, as I now know, though I did not know it then. To frequent the woods from motives of mere utility is mere occupation, and all the feeling raised by it is connected with business. With this I also was well acquainted, for I was often sent to search for a tree or sapling for some special purpose, as, to make a helve [handle of a tool] or a basket or a bottom chair or to make a broom. But an excursion in spring to gather flowers was a very different affair. I am unable to analyze the emotions with which these excursions raised in me but the pleasure on finding a new flower was most decided. The Claytonias, Pulmonaries, Phloxes, Trilliums, and Fringillarias, whose annual reappearance I had greeted in each succeeding spring of my boyhood, were my favorite subjects of botanical investigation later in life.

Summer had its charm not less than spring. Its flowers, its luxuriant herbage, its blackberries and wild cherries, its endless variety of green leaves, its deep and cool shade, with bright gleams of sunshine, its sluggish and half dried brooks, of which, like other boys, I would lie down and drink, and then turn over the flat stones, to see if there were any crawfish beneath.

We may see in the series of autumnal events the care with which God has provided for the preservation of perpetuation of the forest races, by an endless multiplication of germs, and their dependents on the parent tree for life: on its leaves for protection, and the influence of air, to them the "breath of life"; thus illustrating, in the midst of surpassing beauty and solemn grandeur, the relations of child and parent, and showing all to be the workmanship of one wise and Almighty Hand. Such are some of the autumnal lessons taught in the great schoolhouse of the woods.

Pioneer Life in Kentucky: A Series of Reminiscential Letters from Daniel Drake, M.D., of Cincinnati to His Children. Edited by Charles D. Drake. Cincinnati: Robert Clark & Co., 1870. 120–122.

READER REFLECTION

1. *Imagination is a source of fertile fruit for people. What stimulates your imagination? Do you take time to cultivate and utilize your imagination in your life?*
2. *Do you agree that exciting your imagination brings refreshment? A useful way to reenergize yourself? Are there places you go to do so?*

✠ 1.11 The Books That Shape Us

Of our own library I have already spoken incidentally. The family Bible, *Rippon's Hymns*, *Watts' Hymns for Children*, *The Pilgrim's Progress*, and old *Romance of the Days of Knight Errantry*, primers, with a plate representing John Rogers at the stake, spelling books, an arithmetic, and a new almanac for the new year, composed all that I can recollect. When I was 12 or 13 years old, father purchased of a neighbor a copy of *Love's Surveying*, which I still remember afforded me great pleasure. Another book which fell into my hands was [William] Guthrie's *Grammar of Geography*. I feel grateful to Mr. Guthrie for his patient teachings of so dull a pupil, and would like to meet him again.

Before I fell in with the *Grammar of Geography*, I was advanced from [Thomas] Dilworth's to [Noah] Webster's spelling book. I was greatly interested in the new and hard words, and in the new reading it afforded me. A couple of years, or thereabouts, before leaving home, I got *Entick's* [pocket] *Dictionary*, which was of course a great acquisition. I also obtained [William] Scott's lessons [in elocution], which afforded me such new reading, and I used to speak pieces from it at Master Smith's school, when I went to him the second time. In addition (but not to my school library), father purchased I remember (when I was 12 or 13) the *Prompter* [a periodical], *Aesop's Fables*, *Franklin's Life*—all sterling books for boys. A puzzle growing out of the last was his being called Dr., when he had not studied medicine!

Occasionally, father borrowed books for me of Dr. Goforth. Once he brought me the *Farmer's Letters*, a work by [John] Dickinson. Much of it was above my comprehension. Another book from the same source was *Lord Chesterfield's Letters* to his son, inculcating politeness. This fell in mighty close with my tastes, and not less with those of father and mother, who cherished as high and pure an idea of the duty of good breeding as any people on earth. *The Life of Robinson Crusoe* was among my early readings. I have not read it for 45 or 50 years, but long often threatened to do it yet. From the size, it must have been an abridgment that I read in days of yore, but it was so well executed that the whole to me was a living reality.

As to my actual attainments in learning, they were certainly quite limited, and yet I could read and examine a dictionary for the meaning of words, and here is the starting point of all improvement.

Pioneer Life in Kentucky: A Series of Reminiscential Letters from Daniel Drake, M.D., of Cincinnati to His Children. Edited by Charles D. Drake. Cincinnati: Robert Clark & Co., 1870. 163, 164, 166, 167, 169, 172.

READER REFLECTION

1. *What books have been formative for you?*

2. *Drake's fascination with words was lifelong. Reading a book with a dictionary nearby was his method to grow his extensive vocabulary. Once he understood the meaning of a word he never appeared to lose it. Consider exercises to grow your current vocabulary. What value is there in continuing to grow your vocabulary? Is it the starting point of all improvement?*

3. *Recitation or reading of passages allowed Drake to develop his early oratory style. In your work do you have opportunity to develop your oral presentations skills? How important are those skills in your future career?*

⊠ 1.12 ACQUIRE THE FUNDAMENTALS OF LEARNING

The general rule as to my going to school was, to attend in winter, and stay at home for work the other parts of the year, but this was not rigidly observed. I have mentioned the names of McQuitty, Wallace, and Curry, as my teachers till I was nine years old. Father then removed from the village and my schooling was suspended. At the time it was broken off, I had luckily learned to read, and had begun to write. Thus, I was able to make some progress at home.

In a year or two after our removal of a small log schoolhouse was erected by the joint labor of several neighbors. The first teacher, who wielded the hickory mace in this academy, was Jacob Beaden. His function was to teach spelling, reading, writing, and ciphering as far as the rule of three, beyond which he could not go. My next schoolmaster was Kenyon, a Yankee! At that time an *avis rara*, in Kentucky. Under him I made some progress. Continuing to cipher, I reached the "Double Rule of Three" and came at length to a sum which neither of us could work. Of grammar, geography, and definitions, I presume he knew nothing. Still he was of superior scholarship to Beaden. Sometime afterwards I returned for a while to the old sylvan Academy, which now had a new Domino—Master Smith. With him, I began my classical studies. True, he knew nothing of grammar, etymology, geography, mathematics, but he had picked up a dozen lines of Latin poetry, which I had an ambition to commit to memory. I was much taken with the sounds of the words—the first I ever heard beyond my native tongue. From the few I now recollect, I presume the quotation was from the eclogues of Virgil. Master Smith changed his locality, and another long vacation ensued.

My next and last tutor before beginning the study of medicine was my old Master Smith, who now ruled the boys and girls in another log schoolhouse, under a great shell-bark hickory among the haw trees. To him I was sent, more or less, through the spring, summer, and early autumn of the year 1800, when I was in my 15th year. As my destiny to the profession of medicine was now a "fixed fact," I was taking the finishing touches; and yet spelling, reading, writing, and cyphering constituted the curriculum of Master Smith's College.

Pioneer Life in Kentucky: A Series of Reminiscential Letters from Daniel Drake, M.D., of Cincinnati to His Children. Edited by Charles D. Drake. Cincinnati: Robert Clark & Co., 1870. 143, 144, 145, 152, 154, 157, 158.

READER REFLECTION

1. Drake's formal schooling was often interrupted, and even when he was able to attend, the schools had mediocre teachers. By age nine he was able to read, and, later, armed with a dictionary, he could teach himself. Thus, self-learning was foundational for Drake beginning at a young age. Taking the initiative to learn on one's own is fundamental to scholarship and personal growth. How much effort do you put into self-learning?

2. How important is it to continue the process of self-learning after your formal schooling is over and you are out in the "real world"?

⚔ 1.13 LEARN TO DEFEND YOURSELF

Two incidents...remain in my memory, and I will mention them as illustrating my character at that time. A boy by the name of Walter, from mere mischief (for we had a quarrel), struck me a hard blow and cut one of my lips, which I did not resent, as most boys would have done; but quietly put up with it. When I went home at night, and was asked the cause of the assault, father blamed and shamed me for my cowardice. I felt mortified, but was not aroused to any kind or degree of revenge.

The other incident was this. In the open field in which the school house stood, the boys were accustomed to roll great balls of snow, and then dividing themselves into two parties, one was to have possession of the mass, and the other try to take it from them. On one of these occasions, when I belonged to the former battalion, the battle waxed hot enough to melt all the snow on the field. But it was, in fact, a little softer already, and hence our balls were hard and heavy. With these missiles we came to very close quarters, and the small boys, like myself, were sorely pelted on the head and face by the larger. However, I never thought of flinching, and if it had come to fists, feet, and teeth, I am quite certain I should have fought until placed *hors de combat* by some overpowering confusion...

Now how are these two displays of character to be reconciled? They appear to stand in direct opposition. As they involve principles which have run through my whole life, I will offer you my speculations concerning them. Naturally, I took no pleasure in witnessing a combat of any kind, not even that of dogs or gamecocks, the fights of which were in those days, common amusements. The fights of men, which I often saw, also affected me unpleasantly. Thus, I had not the pugnacious temper. Again, I was rather slow to anger, that is, to the point of resentment. Again, mother had taught me to regard fighting as wicked, and had not established in my mind any distinction between fighting in aggression and fighting in defense. She was, *in extenso*, a noncombatant. Finally, when not adequately aroused, I was timid, and the aggressions which are so often productive of fights among boys did not arouse me. The opposite of emotion counteracted my anger. In the snowballing my ambition, not my anger, was up. I was under an adequate motive, one which excited me, and no fear or thought of personal danger came into my mind.

I will illustrate this subject by an incident which occurred about four years afterward, in the early period of my studies with Dr. Goforth. I had a fellow student, and two boys from a neighboring town were boarding and lodging at the doctor's, to go to school. The older and largest, corresponding to me in age and size, offered me various insults, and spoke against me behind my back, but at the time of giving insults I did not resent them. At length, one morning, when the other two had gone downstairs, and we were partly dressed (for we all lodged in the same room), it came into my mind and heart to whip him, although he had not then said a word to me. So at it we went, and in a half a minute he cried out enough! a cry which I should not have uttered by the next morning: and still he would have fought at any time under provocation which would not have moved me to retaliation, but perhaps made me afraid.

Pioneer Life in Kentucky: A Series of Reminiscential Letters from Daniel Drake, M.D., of Cincinnati to His Children. Edited by Charles D. Drake. Cincinnati: Robert Clark & Co., 1870. 155–157.

1. *One of Drake's lifelong approaches to conflict was fighting back when he felt personally attacked or if, on principle, he believed another person to be in error. In such instances he was very passionate, resolute, and sharp-tongued. This position often got him into trouble with colleagues and others. What is your personal response to provocation? Does it serve you well?*

2. *How should a person respond when personally attacked during their career? How can conflicts be resolved when there are disagreements?*

🏵 1.14 RECOGNIZE PERSONAL DEFICIENCIES AND WORK TO ELIMINATE THEM

When I went to master Smith the second time, I felt more than I had ever done before, the necessity of application. I felt anxious concerning the future, knew that my deficiencies were great, and really sought to make the most of my time.

You may ask, how I could know of deficiencies in my preparation for the study of medicine, the science of which I was so ignorant? My answer is at hand, and will involve a notice of my cousin Dr. John Drake.

He was the younger son of uncle Abraham Drake, the tavern keeper, merchant, and rich man of the family. John was five to seven years older than myself. When I was 4 or 5 he used to excite my wonder and that of the other children, with stories of *Jack the Giant-Killer*, *Bluebeard*, and other great men, for which he had a remarkable talent. From the number of his classical books, now in my possession, I infer that he had been sent to school in Washington [Cincinnati] to some good scholar who might have been there. He went to the study of medicine in that town with Dr. Goforth, about the year 1795 or 1796. His progress as a medical student was rapid. His talents were various. In the Thespian Corps he maintained a high rank, and in the debating society his eloquence was enviable. In manners he attained to ease and grace. His person was rather small and delicate, but his presence, I will recollect, was highly prepossessing. In the autumn of 1798 or 1799 he went to Philadelphia to attend lectures, and when I did the same thing in the fall of 1805, and wrote my name on Professor [Benjamin] Barton's register, he immediately inquired after my namesake, and spoke of him in high terms. That the professor should have remembered him so long depressed my spirits, for I felt how greatly behind him I must be; seeing that the idea of being thus remembered could not be entertained by me for a moment. John spent the spring and summer at home in Mayslick with his father, diligently pursuing his studies, and I believe, adding the Latin language to the medical sciences. He was to attend lectures the following winter, and then establish himself in Mayslick, when I was to become his pupil. Now it was from him, in various conversations, and from looking into his classical and medical books, that I came to an apprehension of my inadequate preparation for the enterprise on which I was about to enter. His constitution was frail, and in the month of July he was seized with a slow fever of the typhus kind. The physicians of Washington, Drs. Johnson and Duke, attended him; but he gradually got worse. At length his father, who doted on him, dispatched our cousin Jacob Drake to Cincinnati for Dr. Goforth; but the doctor could not come; and about the time Jacob got back, riding all night, through a tremendous and awful thunderstorm, with some advice in his pocket, John expired; and his remains now repose in the old village churchyard. A young man of the brightest genius and the noblest qualities of heart, he would have conferred distinction on our name; and his memory should be transmitted in the family. All his books and manuscripts came into and remain in my possession.

Pioneer Life in Kentucky: A Series of Reminiscential Letters from Daniel Drake, M.D., of Cincinnati to His Children. Edited by Charles D. Drake. Cincinnati: Robert Clark & Co., 1870. 158–161.

READER REFLECTION

1. *Having role models is an important formative experience for us growing up. Who were/are your role models? What have you learned from them?*
2. *How can you become aware of your own deficiencies, or areas for improvement? Develop a plan to close the gap and turn them into strengths.*

⊠ 1.15 HOW SERENDIPITY DIRECTS OUR LIVES

Had Dr. John Drake lived, I should not have gone to Cincinnati to study medicine, and of a consequence never resided there. In fact, humanly speaking, my whole course of life might have been entirely different from what it has been. I should probably have become a country doctor and a member of the General assembly! His death did not turn father aside from the determination that I should study physic [medicine], and I still continued to make my way daily through two miles of woods to the log School-house on the banks of the Shannon. We had, however, a great deal of work to do on the farm, and I felt that as I was not only soon to leave father, but become an expense to him, I ought to tax myself to the upmost. Thus, I rose early and worked in the field till breakfast time, and after that very commonly *ran* the 2 miles, to be in time. But my health was good, my endurance great, and we always retired early at night.

Pioneer Life in Kentucky: A Series of Reminiscential Letters from Daniel Drake, M.D., of Cincinnati to His Children. Edited by Charles D. Drake. Cincinnati: Robert Clark & Co., 1870. 161.

Reader Reflection

1. *What seems like a small turn of events can turn out to have a major impact on the course of a person's life. Periodically record your life path and identify the small, yet important events that seem like serendipity.*
2. *Do you have the capacity to see the opportunity that presents itself along life's way and adapt creatively while keeping a sense of your life's larger purpose?*

1.16 Responsibility Grows Us

In the midst of this last effort, however, a family affliction arose, which greatly interrupted my studies. Father got a severe injury on his foot, which partially mortified, and three or four of the children were taken down with the ague [malaria] and fever—the first time that that disease had ever visited us. In my letter two years ago, I must have mentioned these facts, but probably did not tell you (boastingly) that when the care of everything turned on mother and myself, my heart grew big with the emotions which such calamities naturally inspire, and with the feeling of responsibility that was quite as natural, producing in my actions their proper fruit; and father and mother commended me for my labors, both indoors and out. To speak of the whole matter frankly, I look back, even from this distant point of time, 47 years, to my conduct with approbation and pleasure. What a precious reward (referring to this life only) there is and striving to do what trying occasions require of us!

Pioneer Life in Kentucky: A Series of Reminiscential Letters from Daniel Drake, M.D., of Cincinnati to His Children. Edited by Charles D. Drake. Cincinnati: Robert Clark & Co., 1870. 161, 162.

Reader Reflection

1. *Responsibility is a great teacher. Think of a time you came upon unexpected responsibility, and record the ways in which you responded positively. What did you learn about yourself from that experience?*

2. *Seek out or volunteer for responsibility early in your career. Do you have some need in your organization that someone needs to step up and take on? In what ways might you grow from it?*

⊠ 1.17 Learn Deeply Instead of Superficially

Childhood is the epoch of mutability, in which impressions rapidly succeed and supersede each other. Children do not dwell long enough on any object, or group of objects, to acquire correct and ascertained ideas of their properties and relations, and hence they investigate badly. This propensity to pass from subject to subject is a principle of our nature; and is designed to introduce us to a first interview with the multitude of surrounding objects, with which it is the business of after life to become more intimately acquainted. But like every other principle of action, it requires control and discipline. Appertaining, as we have seen, especially to childhood and youth, it belongs to a good education to keep it subordinate in manhood. Those in whom this is neglected grow up deficient in habits of protracted investigation, and seldom dwell long enough on any subject to comprehend it fully. Such persons may be styled adult children, and the number is not a few. Gazing for a moment on the superficies of many objects, but looking into the deep structure of none, they seldom perceive the truth, as in most cases, it lies far beneath the surface.

"Causes of Error in the Medical and Physical Sciences." In *Practical Essays on Medical Education in the Medical Profession in the United States.* Cincinnati: Roff & Young, 1832. 72–73.

Reader Reflection

1. *How does a person develop the "habit of protracted investigation" in a learning environment that has a smorgasbord of visual and auditory stimuli?*

2. *What is the utility of possessing the capacity of "protracted investigation" [sustained concentration and study]?*

✠ 1.18 Acquire a Worldview

The Universe is an empire, and God is its sovereign... The different objects which compose the universe are not at rest, nor do they remain in the same relation. Motion is the condition in which most of those on the earth's surface exist; the mass itself is in motion, and even the sun turns on its axis; the other planets of the solar system, have the same movements with ours. It is probable, that the constellation to which our sun belongs, has a progressive motion in the heavens; and, if this is the fact, we may suppose that the whole—the entire universe, is in action. Such being the probability, and in reference to our earth and its productions, the actual fact, it follows, that a state of chaos would sooner or later arise, unless these complicated movements were made on some kind of system. But the experience of the human race in past times, and every day's observation, convince us, that disorder is not the consequence of this action, and, of course, there must be laws of motion; and we believe that God, who made the worlds and all who inhabit them, is the great law-giver. To regulate the revolutions of the planets, he has enacted laws; to guide the action of atoms of matter on other atoms, he has made other laws; to direct the arrangement of those atoms in organized bodies; he has established other laws; and, lastly, to govern man, he has made others, which refer both to this mind and body. Thus, every movement, from that of a satellite round the earth, to the revolution of the sun on its axis; from the rise and fall of a particle of dust, or the growth of a blade of grass, to the voluntary actions of man himself, is regulated by laws, which only God can modify or repeal. The government, then, of the entire universe, is a government of laws, and without them, it would stand still, speedily run into confusion.

"Discipline: Discourse on the Philosophy of Family, School, and College Discipline." *Transactions of the Fourth Annual Meeting of the Western Literary Institute and College of Professional Teachers.* Cincinnati: Josiah Drake Publisher, 1835. 31–32.

Reader Reflection

1. *Can you articulate your worldview (a philosophy of life, how you understand the human condition, and beliefs about the larger universe, how it is organized and your place in it)?*
2. *How does this influence how you live?*

✠ 1.19 Learn from Your First Illness Experience

The first illness I remember (and the only one in those days), was, indeed, both severe and protracted. It arose from a fall, on the ice I think, and produced an inflammation with fever on the lower part of the spine. It terminated in an abscess, and an ulcer that continued for a long time. I was attended by Dr. Goforth, and distinctly remember how anxious I used to feel for his visits, and, at the same time, how much I dreaded his probe. On the voyage down the river, he and my father had become, as the saying is, sworn friends. Father thought him on many points a very weak man, and knew that he was intemperate, but believed him a great physician. Already, when five years old, I had been promised to him as a student; and among the remembrances of that period is my being called "Dr. Drake." No wonder, then, as nearly sixty years have rolled away, that I sometimes have a difficulty in passing myself off for the old and primary Dr. Drake.

Pioneer Life in Kentucky: A Series of Reminiscential Letters from Daniel Drake, M.D., of Cincinnati to His Children. Edited by Charles D. Drake. Cincinnati: Robert Clark & Co., 1870. 26, 27.

Reader Reflection

1. *Consider your first memories of being ill. What did you learn from that experience, or additional illness experiences, about human life?*

✠ 1.20 Deciding on Your Career

The long talked of project—that of "making me a doctor," had at length been finally settled in the affirmative. I was to enter on the study in a few months with my cousin, Dr. John Drake, whose education was then nearly completed, and whose genius was only equaled by his great moral purity. With this prospect before me, he was taken ill in July with typhus fever, and died in August. This was my first disappointment, and a real misfortune to me, for he would have been a good preceptor, and I could've studied at home, and thus saved father an expense which he was in no way prepared to meet. He courageously persevered, however, in his cherished purpose, and I had to submit, although on his account I would've preferred being bound to a trades man, and had actually selected a master, Mr. Stout, of Lexington, a sadler, to whom some of my cornfield companions had already gone.

But my preparatory education was not yet completed. As a reader, I was equal to any in what I regarded as the highest perfection, a loud and tireless voice. In chirography [handwriting] I was so-so, in geography obscure, and in history, zero. In arithmetic, I had gone as far as the double rule of three, practice, tare and tret, interest, and even a fraction in decimals. My greatest acquirement, that of which I was rather proud, was my knowledge of Surveying, acquired from Love [John Love, *The Art of Surveying and Measuring the Land Made Easy*], but which I have long since forgotten. Of grammar I knew nothing, and unfortunately there was no one within my reach who could teach it.

Meanwhile other arrangements were making for the life before me, such as knitting socks, making course India muslin shirts instead of tow linen, providing a couple of cotton pocket handkerchiefs, and purchasing a white roram [wool and fur] hat.

Father visited Dr. Goforth in Cincinnati and on his return, announced that all was arranged, and that I was to go down before the setting in of winter. I was to live in the Doctor's family, and he was to pay $400, provided I remain, as it was expected I would, four years, by which time, I was to be transmitted into a doctor, as I should then be 19! My whole time, however, was not to be given up to the study of medicine, for the doctor was to send me to School for two quarters, that I might learn Latin. But as was sagely decided, it was not to be done *before* I begin the study of medicine, but at some future time.

I was fond of study, but not passionately so, and if I had any aspirations, they were not intense, and several circumstances conspired to countervail them. First, I had looked into the medical books of my cousin, and found them so learned, technical, and obscure, that I was convinced my education was too limited. Second, my father was too poor to pay for what he had undertaken, and was too ailing to dispense with my labors on the farm. Third, I was a great homebody; never been out of the family more than a day or night at a time; felt timid about going among strangers into town, and mingling with the "quality." Finally I was the distressed at the idea of an absence of 4 to 5 or five months. At length, all arrangements were made.

The morning of 16 December 1800 at length arrived, and the parting came with it. Lizzy was 13, Lydia 10, Ben six, Lavinia three or four, and Livingston about one. There we all were in the cabin where more than half had been born, where I had carried the younger ones in my arms, and amused them with the good old cow brindle, as she drank her slop at the door while mother milked her. The parting over, we mounted, and I took a farewell look at the little cabin, then wiped my eyes.

Pioneer Life in Kentucky: A Series of Reminiscential Letters from Daniel Drake, M.D., of Cincinnati to His Children. Edited by Charles D. Drake. Cincinnati: Robert Clark & Co., 1870. 229, 230, 232, 233, 235, 236.

READER REFLECTION

1. *What influence did your family have on your decision about leaving home or choosing your career path? How did you manage your feelings about these decisions? Is there a right way to deal with these feelings? Also, consider what character qualities are needed to be successful in these situations.*

2. *How did you decide on your career? As you started your career did you have some hesitation or concerns about your ability to succeed at it? Is this common? How should a person manage these feelings?*

✠ 1.21 PARENTAL EXPECTATIONS AND SACRIFICES

In the long period from youth to age, I had my trials and troubles, it is true, but it is in a stage of transition from one state of society to another, from the rural to the civic, from the rude to the refined, from obscurity to notoriety. The *caste* to which I belonged was to be changed; and in the arrangements of Providence, I was made, unconsciously, the instrument by which that changed was to be effected. The conception of this change was less my own than my father's. He was a gentleman by nature, and a Christian from convictions produced by simple and unassisted study of the word of God. His poverty he regretted; his ignorance he deplored. His natural instincts were to knowledge, refinement, and honorable influence in the affairs of the world. In consulting the traditions of the family he found no higher condition than his own as their lot in past times; but he had formed a conception of something more elevated and resolved on its attainment; not for himself and mother, nor for all his children—for either would have been impossible—but for some member of the family. He would make a beginning; he would set his face toward the land of promise, although, like Moses, he himself would never enter it. Imperfectly as I have fulfilled this destiny which, under the arrangements of Providence, he assigned to me, I cannot doubt that if he and mother should be permitted to look down upon the family group to whom you will read this epistle, they would gratefully exclaim, "The cherished desire of our hearts will at last be gratified."

Pioneer Life in Kentucky: A Series of Reminiscential Letters from Daniel Drake, M.D., of Cincinnati to His Children. Edited by Charles D. Drake. Cincinnati: Robert Clark & Co., 1870. 98–99.

READER REFLECTION

1. *How have parental expectations shaped you? Have their expectations been fulfilled?*
2. *What sacrifices did your parents make for you so that you might have a better life than they?*

⊞ 1.22 BEGINNING MY MEDICAL APPRENTICESHIP

Beginning on 20 December 1800, at Peach Grove where the Lytle house now stands, my first assigned duties were to read [John] Quincy's *Dispensatory* and grind quicksilver into *unguentum mercurial* [mercury ointment]; the latter of which from previous practice on a Kentucky hand mill I found much easier of the two... New studies and a new studio awaited me; and through the ensuing spring and summer the adjoining meadow with its forest shade trees,... Underneath those shade trees,...it was my allotted task to commit to memory [William] Cheselden on the Bones and [John] Innes on the Muscles, without specimens of the former or plates of the latter; and afterwards to meander the currents of Humoral pathology, of [Herman] Boerhaave and [Gerard] Van Swieten; without having studied the Chemistry of [Jean-Antoine] Chaptal, the Physiology of [Albrecht] von Haller, or the Materia Medica of [William] Cullen.

Such was the beginning of medical education in Cincinnati. I said beginning, for I was its first pupil. I've already mentioned the aversion of my preceptor to the system of Dr. [Benjamin] Rush; which went so far, that he forbade my reading the writings of the gentleman which he happened to have. The new publications, brought out by Dr. [John] Stites, were, however, a temptation to disobedience not be resisted and before my master was aware of this fact, I commanded his respect, by knowing things of which his prejudices have kept him ignorant.

You will smile when I tell you that a consequence of this was, that he who never saw defects in one he loved, soon after this—in 1803—begin to ask my opinion on cases which he took me with him to see. In the spring the following year, he made me his partner; in the summer the next, when I was preparing to visit the University [of] Pennsylvania, he favored me with an autograph diploma, setting forth my ample attainment, in all the branches of the profession; and subscribing himself, as he really was, Surgeon General of the First Division of the Ohio militia. This was undoubtedly the first medical diploma ever granted in the interior valley of North America.... By its authority I practiced medicine for the next 11 years; at which time it was corroborated by another from the University [of Pennsylvania]—the first ever conferred, by that or any other school on a Cincinnati student.

"Early Physicians, Scenery, and Society of Cincinnati." In *Discourses Delivered by Appointment before the Cincinnati Medical Library Association.* Cincinnati: Moore and Anderson, 1852.

READER REFLECTION

1. *What motivates you to master information you find challenging? Hypothesize what were the great motivators for Drake to learn—what could have driven him to do this? Do you have some of these motivators?*
2. *Can gaining knowledge, beyond that of your teacher, open doors of opportunity?*

✖ 1.23 LESSONS FROM A MENTOR

Dr. William Goforth, of whom I know more than all of who have been mentioned, was born in the city of New York 1766. His preparatory education was what may be called tolerably good.... [A]round 1787 he and the other students of the forming school of New York City were disbursed by a mob, raised against the cultivators of anatomy. He at once resolved to accompany his brother-in-law, the late Gen. John S. Gano, into the west; and on 10 June 1788 landed at Maysville, Kentucky, then called Limestone. Settling in Washington, 4 miles from the river, then in population the second town of Kentucky, he soon acquired great popularity and had the chief business of the county for 11 years.

Fond of change, he determined to leave [Washington]; and in 1799 reached Columbia, where his father, Judge Goforth, one of the earliest and most distin-guished pioneers of Ohio, resided. In the spring of the next year 1800 he removed to Cincinnati, and occupied the Peach-Grove house, vacated by Dr. Allison's removal to the country. Bringing with him a high reputation, having an influential family connection, being the successor of Dr. Allison, he immediately acquired an extensive practice. But without these advantages he would have gotten business, for on the whole, he had the most winning manners of any physician I ever knew. Yet they were all his own, for in deportment he was quite an original. The painstaking and respectful courtesy with which he treated the poorest and humblest people of the village seemed to secure their gratitude; and the more especially as he dressed with precision, and never left his house in the morning till his hair was powdered by our itinerant barber, John Arthurs, and his gold-headed cane was grasped by his gloved hand. His kindness of heart was as much a part of his nature, as his hair powder was of his costume; and what might not be given through benevolence, could always be extracted by flattery, coupled with professions of friendship, and the sincerity of which he never questioned. In conversation he was precise yet fluent, and abounded in anecdotes which he told in a way that others could not imitate. He took a warm interest in the politics what was then the North Western territory, being at all times the earnest advocate of popular rights. His devotion to Masonry, then a cherished institution of the village, was such that he always embellished his signature with some of its emblems. His handwriting was peculiar, but so remarkably plain that his poor patients felt flattered to think he should have taken so much pain in writing for *them*. This part of his character, many of us might find a useful example.... [L]ooking back to its results, I may say, that in all, except the most acute forms of disease, his success was creditable to his sagacity and tact.

"Early Physicians, Scenery, and Society of Cincinnati." In *Discourses Delivered by Appointment before the Cincinnati Medical Library Association.* Cincinnati: Moore and Anderson, 1852.

Reader Reflection

1. *Identify the character qualities of Dr. Goforth that Drake recalled nearly fifty years later.*
2. *Who were/are your mentors? What valuable lessons have they shared with you? What have you learned from the way they practiced their craft?*

⬗ 1.24 Become Self-Aware and Learn to Appreciate What Motivates You to Achieve

I was free from gross vices, or even a tendency to them, and was protected by some degree of conscientiousness. I was still further defined by love of approbation and praise, which was far from being either dilute or easily clogged; but I was not made vain, self conceited, or a spoiled child by its administration. On the contrary, the pleasure it afforded was mingled with a kind of regret that I did not deserve more of the same savory element of the soul, and every new resolution to earn additional supplies by greater exertions in the line of duty. This was a salutary effect of commendation and indicated a low state of pride. That passion was, indeed, never strong; and, moreover, was counterpoised by humility which always suggested how far short I came of the excellence which ought to be attained. With these traits, if I had been born a slave, I should never have become a rebel, but conforming to my condition, rendering diligent service, have acquired the confidence of my master. I had patience without apathy, and endurance without insensibility. My curiosity was keen, and my desire for knowledge much stronger than my consciousness of a capacity for acquiring it. I thought how pleasant it would be to know a great deal; but dared not hope that my talents would procure for me the gratification. I had an idea that those who have studied science deeply, and written books, or became otherwise distinguished, had not only been favored with greater opportunities, but far greater talents than myself. As to my actual attainments in learning, they were certainly quite limited, yet I could read and examine a dictionary for the meaning of words; and here is the starting point of all improvement. My intellectual preparation consisted less, perhaps, in my actual scholarship, then in the want of those habits of sustained application and the strength of memory which (in ordinary minds) can only be acquired in boyhood. I had, it is true, an ability to engage readily in any study, but, at the same time, might be easily diverted from it to any other. I had not been disciplined into the constancy of attention which it is an office of the school master to establish within the walls of the school, where nature, my greatest teacher, is shut out. Now, as nature teaches by the works and events which, in the embodiment, constitute the best definition of the word itself, it follows, from her complex character, that her pupils are instructed in many things at the same time or in quick succession, and that, although the faculty of observation, from continued exercise, may acquire much strength, the attention is not drilled into concentrated protracted devotion to one subject. It results, then, from all I have said, that when I engage in the study of medicine, I had a natural and acquired preparation to become a useful physician, but not to enlarge the boundaries of medical science, by the discoveries and inventions of genius.

Pioneer Life in Kentucky: A Series of Reminiscential Letters from Daniel Drake, M.D., of Cincinnati to His Children. Edited by Charles D. Drake. Cincinnati: Robert Clark & Co., 1870. 171, 172, 173.

Reader Reflection

1. How do you think your early experiences of learning have shaped your interests and talents?

2. What are your chief motivators that drive accomplishment?

LEAVING A LEGACY

✠ 1.25 Seek to Develop Your Intellect and Character

My young friends! As one star differeth from another star in glory though not in the purity of its light, so some of you will be more brilliant than others in the light of intellect, but all may be equal in pureness of heart and propriety of life, elements of character without which no intellectual energy ever bestowed true greatness! Without moral purity, mental endowments raise man into a monster to be gazed at from a distance but never approached as a friend or benefactor! The high and rocky mountain is an object of admiration from below, but no one fixes his abode on its cold and stormy battlements—the hills and valleys, which smile around its base, have fertility of soil, and from their warm bosom, send up the corn which nourishes and the herb that heals.

"The Formation of Professional Character" [1835]. In *Frontiersman of the Mind,* edited by Charles D. Aring. Cincinnati: History of the Health Sciences Library and Museum, University of Cincinnati, 1985.

Reader Reflection

1. *Intellect and character are not the same. What do you mean when you talk about each? How do you develop both? Discuss how necessary they are to create a meaningful legacy.*

✠ 1.26 Cultivate Punctuality and Patience

Mold yourselves to habits of punctuality and patience. Sickness renders men impatient and irritable, women patient but sensitive in deference to your attention. In the practice of Medicine, the interests and feelings of the sick will not permit them to pardon your neglect. They cannot always distinguish between the dangerous and the trifling, and when they send for the physician they expect to see him at the appointed time. But, if he has not formed habits and cherished principles of punctuality in youth, he will not practice it successfully in age. I am aware that in no profession is it more difficult to be punctual; but on that very account is it the more necessary to cultivate the habit within that period of life when character is in its forming stage.

"The Formation of Professional Character" [1835]. In *Frontiersman of the Mind,* edited by Charles D. Aring. Cincinnati: History of the Health Sciences Library and Museum, University of Cincinnati, 1985.

READER REFLECTION

1. How is punctuality related to success? How important is punctuality in working with others?

2. What method(s) can be used to stay punctual?

✦ 1.27 TRAIN DELIBERATELY FOR CHARACTER

Cherish feelings of benevolence and humanity. It is in early life only that they can be cultivated. When they are required in the practice of medicine, you may not be able to call them to your aid, if you have allowed them to slumber unexercised in the deep and unfrequented caverns of your heart. Ambition, cupidity, and selfishness in the progress of years will choke them, if they be not trained and invigorated, as tender and sensitive plants are overgrown and buried up by thorns and thistles when the ground is not cultivated. We have many examples of striking similarity between the laws of body and mind and here is one. You may use and discipline the eye in childhood and youth, till it will acquire a governing influence among the organs of sense, and in like manner you may exercise and stimulate any one of the sentiments or propensities of the soul, till it will mount above the rest, or neglecting its proper use suffer it to languish in worthless inferiority.

"The Formation of Professional Character" [1835]. In *Frontiersman of the Mind,* edited by Charles D. Aring. Cincinnati: History of the Health Sciences Library and Museum, University of Cincinnati, 1985.

READER REFLECTION

1. Discuss: training for character is better done early in life than later as an adult.

2. Do you have an approach to discipline and train your senses? How do you train your "sentiments or propensities of the soul"?

✦ 1.28 BE INDUSTRIOUS—BUILD YOUR CAPACITY FOR WORK

The first object of every student should be to form a love and habit of Industry. No occupation in society calls for greater industry than the Medical. The senses must be active, the feelings must be active, the intellect must be active, the body must be active. Without industry, the facts and principles of the Science cannot be acquired, the duties of the profession cannot be discharged, conscience cannot be satisfied, fortune cannot be accumulated, fame cannot be won.

Action is the law of the universe. It is not less the law of the little universe, the microcosm—Man. There is no efficiency, no sound professional health and excellence, no onward movement, no ascent, no unfolding, no conversion of the dawn into the warm and sweeping tide of summer noon without industry—resolute, sleepless, untiring, unfaltering, uncomplaining industry. How would our mother earth get on if she were not industrious? In this respect, gentlemen, she is a model for all her sons. (I hope you are young enough to be enamoured with feminine models of excellence.) She in fact never sleeps, for while one hemisphere falls into that state, the other is wide awake. I wish gentlemen your cerebral hemispheres were capable of doing this, for while one side of the brain went to sleep under a dull lecture the other could keep awake and listen.

Our good mother earth, moreover, carries on many kinds of business at once, and here again she is worthy of your imitation. She travels round the sun and at the same time turns on her heel. She keeps her blood in perpetual circulation. She breathes in the gale. She casts the hill into the valley, and raises the Continent from the depths of the ocean—covers it with green carpets, enamels it with tufts of flowers, and overshadows it with magnificent trees. The wild animals feed and frolic beneath their spreading branches, and the melody of song-birds floats through all their leafy alcoves.

You are of the earth formed of the clods of the valley, and destined to mingle with them. You live and must die under the dominion of the same great law of nature, with the rest of creation and subject to every penalty attached to its violation. Open your eyes to this momentous fact now while you are yet young, and may form your habits of life. Train yourselves to physical and intellectual labour. Cherish the opinion that inaction begets sluggishness, that stagnation tends to putrefaction, and torpor ends in death.

Your industry should be such as to invigorate your frames and form you for bodily endurance.

"The Formation of Professional Character" [1835]. In *Frontiersman of the Mind*, edited by Charles D. Aring. Cincinnati: History of the Health Sciences Library and Museum, University of Cincinnati, 1985.

1. *Discuss the role of industriousness in leaving a legacy.*

2. *Do you agree that to practice medicine you have to engage your senses, your intellect, your emotions, and your body all at once and over and over again?*

✖ 1.29 THE BENEFITS OF INDUSTRIOUSNESS

Man is an indolent animal. By nature he loves repose. Exertion is a forced state: the offspring of necessity, for the instigation of some passion, more powerful than the love of ease. Children, although constitutionally active in the pursuit of amusement, are averse to labor, and require stimulation and discipline to form habits of industry. I have been amazed to observe, how little fathers and mothers are aware of these truths; or, if aware of them, how little they are governed by the conviction. On this point, admonition is more necessary to the rich and the poor. Among the latter, children are often obliged to work for food and clothing—among the former, it is not uncommon, to see them grow up in ease and idleness. Youth is the era of life in which our habits are formed; and he who grows up in indolence and riches, may live and die in idleness in poverty. When extravagance and dissipation have squandered his inheritance, even the stimulus of want, may not break his established habits. This subject is of such deep interest, to all of us who are parents, that I cannot refrain from dwelling on it a moment longer.

Industry, promotes the health and bodily growth of children: *Indolence*, impairs both.

Industry, renders their studies easy and pleasing: *Indolence*, makes them truants.

Industry, is a substitute for genius: *Indolence*, renders genius ineffective.

Industry, preserves our inheritance: *Indolence*, squanders it away.

Industry, inspire society with confidence: *Indolence*, repels its confidence.

Industry, provides for casualties: *Indolence*, renders us helpless under them.

Industry, makes present provision for old age: *Indolence*, loads it with cares and embarrassment.

Industry, provides for children: *Idleness*, fails to do this and limits their opportunities, blasts their prospects, and, when we die, leaves them dependent on a heartless world.

Industry, gives us the means of charitable and patriotic donation: *Idleness*, prevents our co-operating and works of beneficence, and inflicts on us the character of sordidness.

Industry, contributes to give us long life, while it condenses into a short one, the fruits of many years: *Indolence,* abridges life, and renders the longest unproductive of happy results.

Finally, *Industry,* has transformed this vast and beautiful region, into a cultivated and populous country; so abundant in comforts, and so noble in its public works, that when abroad, one is proud to say, in the matter of an ancient Roman, "I am a citizen of Ohio." *Idleness,* would have left it thinly peopled wilderness, without developed resources, destitute of the arts of civilized life, and inhabited by a few helpless adventurers; still grappling with Indians and beasts of prey, on the very spot where the eminent representatives of a million of freeman, are deliberating on the public good!

An Oration on the Causes, Evils, and Preventives of Intemperance. Columbus: Olmstead & Bailhache, Printers, 1831.

Reader Reflection

1. *How would you assess your own work ethic? Did your early experiences teach you to be industrious? If so, how? (or how not?)*
2. *Reflect on the benefits of industry to accomplish your life goals. Can you draw a linkage between your work effort and achieving your goals?*

1.30 Learn to Be Methodical to Maximize Your Productiveness

But you may have industry and endurance under fatigue and exposure, and yet be unsuccessful in results. *To be productive, your industry must be methodical.* Method involves the idea of an ultimate object, and the contemplation of many things in connection so as to understand their relations to each other and to that object. Immethodical industry is the parent of mere display of bustle and hubbub, of high excitement, flashing from object to object, like the lightnings which in our hot summer nights play among the clouds, but send down no showers of rain to fertilize the earth. Undirected is indeed unproductive effort. Could you double the Cape of Good Hope and reach the glowing and spicy east, by sailing without chart or compass? When you can, and not till then, may you hope without method to reach the fairyland where the winged herald resides, who shall proclaim your achievements to an admiring world.

"The Formation of Professional Character" [1835]. In *Frontiersman of the Mind,* edited by Charles D. Aring. Cincinnati: History of the Health Sciences Library and Museum, University of Cincinnati, 1985.

Reader Reflection

1. *To be productive our work must be goal-directed, and we need to understand the factors that will help achieve that goal. We must also have a map or a compass (a well-defined plan) to reach our goals. Is your work informed by goals and well-thought-out plans?*
2. *How likely is a person to develop a legacy without being goal-directed?*

⊠ 1.31 Cultivate a Meekness of Spirit to Counter Human Pride and Hubris

Meekness of spirit is scarcely a more necessary predisposition for the reception of divine, than scientific truth. The self-sufficient philosopher never inquires into his defects. When he contemplates himself, it is rather to admire his excellences than to correct his imperfections. He views the former with a mote, the later with a beam in his "mind's eye." He employs a mirror, which reflects only the beauties of his character; and should it, at any time, become true to nature, he turns from the unwelcome glimpse of his deformities, as from things to be concealed and forgotten, not corrected. To expose them to society would mortify him still more. He is even reluctant to display his improvements, as they would imply previous defects of knowledge, and approximate him to mortals of a common mold. A student of this class often prefers to remain ignorant, rather than appear so; but it is, especially in advanced life, that pride interferes most fatally with improvement in science. In youth, vanity sometimes tempers this indomitable passion; but in process of time, it not infrequently subdues every opposing sentiment, and, becoming fortified by habit, governs the character of the individual, with the spirit of a tyrant. Hence the obstinate perseverance in ancient errors, the cynical sneering at late discoveries, the dogmatism, the pomp, and the real or affected skepticism, which in medicine so often render old age ridiculous, and sometimes, seriously impede the dissemination of new truths. I know of no cure for this *fungus hematodes* of the mind, when it has become deeply rooted, but in youth it may be eradicated, and every student should seek to cast it out.

"Causes of Error in the Medical and Physical Sciences." In *Practical Essays on Medical Education in the Medical Profession in the United States.* Cincinnati: Roff & Young, 1832. 78.

READER REFLECTION

1. *Do pride and arrogance interfere with building a legacy?*
2. *Do you struggle with pride and arrogance? How does a person maintain a "meekness of spirit" while experiencing success?*
3. *Have you ever seen the consequences of hubris?*

⊠ 1.32 THE VALUE OF AN OBSERVATION ROAD TRIP IN YOUR FORMATIVE YEARS

One of the leading objects of the Western Museum Society [is] to collect and preserve the natural and artificial curiosities of the United States, and especially of that portion which we inhabit. If any enlargement of mind can result from the examination of them one exhibited in the museum, the same affect would be produced, in a much higher degree, by inspecting and contemplating them in their natural situations. I cannot, therefore, but regret, that we do not attach more importance to journeys of observation through our own country. Travels of this kind where eloquently recommended, almost a century ago, by the celebrated Linnaeus, and ought to make a part of the education of every young man. After having completed his scholastic, Academic, or collegiate course, and acquired the rudiments of his trade or profession, he could do nothing so well calculated to enrich his mind with useful knowledge, and qualify him for the practical duties of future life, as to travel through his native land. The objections that preclude the greater number of our young men from foreign traveling cannot lie against domestic, which I do not hesitate to say would be equally serviceable. It is quite deplorable to observe in what utter ignorance of the condition of their native country they usually engage in the career of business that is allotted to them. Whether destined to be farmers, mechanics, or merchants; physicians or divines; soldiers, lawyers, or even politicians or statesman they, in general, enter upon their respective pursuit with equal ignorance of the geography, natural history, and statistics of their theater of action; and of the character and genius of the people with whom all their future relations are to be formed. A few of our sons are sent to Europe; but this, even supposing them to derive some improvement from such a journey, does not make them acquainted with their own country, and cannot, therefore, supersede the necessity of exploring it. Such as rely on foreign journeys only, resemble scholars who spend their lives in the study of Greek and Roman literature and die quite ignorant of their own. Accomplishing much which cannot be condemned, though but little that we can approve, they are to be admired rather than imitated, I would not, however, discourage foreign traveling, but it should be preceded by domestic.

An Anniversary Discourse, On the State and Prospects of the Western Museum Society. Cincinnati: Looker, Palmer, and Reynolds, 1820.

Reader Reflection

1. *Consider taking a journey of observation to learn about the people and the communities in your region or in your nation. Where you will work and provide service?*
2. *What would you want to learn by taking an "observation road trip" of your region? How might these observations help build a legacy?*

1.33 Useful Knowledge as the Basis of Societal Happiness

If we perceive, then, an increase of useful knowledge the true secret of our permanent happiness; if literature can supply the talismanic agent of our prosperity and power, and philosophy, like 'a pillar of fire by night,' direct our wandering footsteps to the temple of glory, let us not ignobly stay our hands from the labors by which, only, philosophy and letters can be made to flourish. Let the architects of our national greatness conform to the dictates of science, and the monuments they construct will rise beautiful as our hills, imperishable as our mountains, and lofty as their summits, which tower sublimely above the clouds.

An Anniversary Discourse, On the State and Prospects of the Western Museum Society. Cincinnati: Looker, Palmer, and Reynolds, 1820.

Reader Reflection

1. *Is an increase in useful knowledge the secret of true happiness? What sort of knowledge contributes to your personal happiness?*
2. *Drake found delight in learning. How does a person develop this delight? How can a delight in learning assist you in your career?*

✠ 1.34 Enjoy a Spouse as Friend, Co-laborer, and Motivator

We [Drake and his wife, Harriet] began the world in love and hope and poverty. It was all before us, and we were under the influence of the same ambition to possess it; to acquire not wealth merely but friends, knowledge, influence, distinction. We had equal industry and equal aspirations. She devoted herself to every duty of her station, and might have been a model to those much older and, in bodily powers, much abler than herself. But her active understanding and warm sensibilities did not suffer her attention to exhaust herself on objects of domestic economy. Her mind was highly inquisitive, and she soon manifested a rising interest in my studies and literary pursuits. She evinced a fondness for my society; even when my attention was absorbed by these objects, it was not long before she became my companion when I was engaged in study. I retired not from the association, and custom soon rendered it desirable. She often read to me select passages from books which attracted to her attention, while I was reading those of a different kind. Her selections were always marked by the good sense and good taste that would characterize her whole life. I read to her in turn, and she comprehended and commented. She seldom wrote, but soon manifested that she was an excellent judge of composition. She not only sat by my side conversing, more or less, while I wrote at various times the most that I have written, but my constant practice was to exhibit to her inspection whatever I wrote. She saw the first drafts, and criticized with taste, judgment, severity, and love. We were thus together personally and spiritually, in most of my domestic hours. When abroad for social enjoyment, we seldom were without each other. I had no separate social or sensual gratifications, no tavern orgies, no political club recreations, no dissipated pleasures nor companions. Society was no society to me without her presence and cooperation.

We lived together, not merely at home and in the houses in society of our friends, but frequented, as far as possible, in conjunction, all places of rational curiosity, of improvement, and of innocent and attractive amusements. On such occasions, her observations were always just, instructive, and piquant. I relied upon her taste and judgment; I adopted her approval; I submitted my own impressions to her decision; I was gratified in proportion as she approved and enjoyed.

"Emotions, Reflections, and Anticipations" [1826 or 1827]. In *Pioneer Life in Kentucky: A Series of Reminiscential Letters from Daniel Drake, M.D., of Cincinnati to His Children.* Edited by Charles D. Drake. Cincinnati: Robert Clark & Co., 1870. xiv–xv.

Reader Reflection

1. *Who are the person(s) in your life who challenge and motivate you to good works?*
2. *How have these relationships grown and matured through time? How have they informed your work?*

1.35 Contrasting Legacies

At that time [1806], when I was but twenty years old, I had mingled little with the world, and probably felt proud of my superior culinary achievements. It seems most likely that no feeling of an opposite kind existed in my bosom, or I should have remembered it; for I do remember one mortification of that voyage [returning from Philadelphia]. When [my traveling party was] approaching Maysville, we began to dress up and prepare for the landing. Each put on his best clothes, and I recollect Dr. Bernard Gaines Farrar, Sr. especially exerted himself, because, as I suppose, he had relatives in the neighborhood of the town. I also put on my best coat, that is, my coat worn on a horseback journey of 18 days in the fall, for four months in Philadelphia, and over the mountains to Pittsburgh in the spring, to say nothing of cooking in it through a flat-boat voyage of ten days. The contrast it made with theirs gave me a feeling of mortification, which I have occasionally recollected since. Could I have looked into the distant future, that feeling would have been annihilated; for I should have discovered that if the morning sun shines more brightly on some, the evening beams of the impartial luminary fall in greater mellowness on others. I should have seen, that forty years afterward, one would be in his grave, after having almost his heart broken by an only child, to whom he could not even venture to bequeath the remnants of an estate which had been squandered on or by that profligate son. I should have seen another retired from his profession with a shattered constitution, and worse spirits, without habits of intellectual cultivation, deprived of his best and oldest children, and falling out of sympathy with the society around; whence his old friends were dropping away one by one, without being replaced by new ones; as the jewels fall from the crown of a decayed monarch, who is too poor to replace them. I have seen the third, as I saw him yesterday, with a wrinkled and sallow face, false hair, and green goggly spectacles, unsettled in place and purpose, his sons in Mexico and California, his wife dead, and not a daughter by birth, marriage, or adoption, to care for and caress him.

Pioneer Life in Kentucky: A Series of Reminiscential Letters from Daniel Drake, M.D., of Cincinnati to His Children. Edited by Charles D. Drake. Cincinnati: Robert Clark & Co., 1870. 105–106.

Reader Reflection

1. *Consider how embarrassment and shame can be motivators. Describe a personal experience that you may have had where the fear of embarrassment or shame influenced your behavior.*
2. *Note the contrast of legacies in these different individuals.*

❖ 1.36 Do Not Rest on the Accomplishments of Your Ancestors

Not having commenced our career in barbarism, we are without the characteristics of an aboriginal nation. Our annals are recorded and uninterrupted. We were detached from civilized portions of the old world, and brought with us the habits of thought and action, the tastes, propensities, and passions, which belong to a refined society. Although a young nation, our people are at maturity in much of what belongs to ancient communities. The edifice is new, but the materials of which it is constructed were previously fashioned and employed elsewhere. We have, therefore, the wants and the desires of a highly civilized condition, while for our acknowledged deficiency in the means of gratifying them, we cannot offer as an apology, that we are a new people. With as little propriety can it be urged, that we suffered a premature alienation from the mother country, for the very act of wisdom and heroism which disjoined us from the parent stock, were indubitable evidence of our being prepared for the separation. These, however, were the exploits of our fathers, and I fear that too much reliance has been placed upon them. Have we not admired the greatness of their achievements when we should have been laboring to perpetuate the blessings of which they are the source? Have not our eyes been dazzled by the splendor of their virtues, until we have sometimes been rendered inseparable to what we must perform to make us worthy of such distinguished ancestors? Have we not too frequently beguiled ourselves with the idea, that the formation and adoption of our federal Constitution, was the full establishment of our Independence? Like children who subsist upon their patrimony, have we not drawn with prodigality upon a heritage of fame and glory, which it was our duty to augment?

An Anniversary Discourse, On the State and Prospects of the Western Museum Society. Cincinnati: Looker, Palmer, and Reynolds, 1820.

READER REFLECTION

1. *Each generation builds on the previous one, and some are fortunate to have great role models and take pride in what they accomplished, but Drake challenges us not to rest on the laurels of prior generations, but rather take up the torch to further or augment what they have done. How does a person avoid the spirit of complacency? How do we make certain that we continue to look forward?*

2. *What must be done to augment/improve upon the work of the previous generation?*

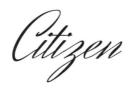

Citizen

"A citizen of exemplary virtue and public spirit"

"He loved to disseminate as well as acquire knowledge, and he loved to disseminate it because of the good it did. This was his public spirit."

—Charles D. Drake, in *Pioneer Life in Kentucky: A Series of Reminiscential Letters from Daniel Drake, M.D., of Cincinnati to His Children*

2.1 *Destiny Is Shaped by Where You Live*

2.2 *A Region's Natural Assets Predict Its Future*

2.3 *Know Your Region's Territory*

2.4 *Recognize the Value of Studying the Natural Resources of a Region*

2.5 *Record for Posterity How Your City Was Named: Cincinnati*

2.6 *City Planning in Cincinnati*

2.7 *Promote the Advantages of Your Community*

2.8 *Know the Ethnic Groups in Your Community*

2.9 *Factors That Shift Community Demographics*

2.10 *Why Ohioans Are Called Buckeyes*

2.11 *Envision an Enduring Community Culture*

2.12 *Reward and Punishment Govern Human Behavior and Are the Foundation of Society*

2.13 *A Universal Principle Providing Safety and Undergirding a Free Society*

2.14 *Take Care of the Poor*

2.15 *Call Out the Consequences of a Bad Law—The Fugitive Slave Act of 1850*

2.16 *Love Is Needed to Address Social Disparities*

2.17 *Recognize the Social Forces Driving Behaviors in the Community*

2.18 *The Value of a Museum Displaying the Great Circle of Knowledge*

2.19   *How a College and a Museum Complement One Another*

2.20   *Study and Memorialize the Past in Your Community*

2.21   *Appreciate, Support, and Promote the Fine Arts*

2.22   *Create a Lecture Series for the Public Good*

2.23   *Promote the Value of Books*

2.24   *Create a Literary Society*

2.25   *The Critical Role of Roads for Enhancing Commerce*

2.26   *Recommended Improvements to Facilitate Community Connections*

2.27   *Proposing and Predicting the Benefits of a Railroad from Cincinnati to Charleston*

2.28   *Why Communities Should Value Medical Schools*

2.29   *Organize Medical Schools to Be under the Sovereign Power of the State and Locally Managed*

2.30   *The Best Clinicians in the Community Should Teach in Medical Schools*

2.31   *Work with the Legislature to Create and Support a Medical College*

2.32   *Create a Teaching Hospital*

2.33   *Recognize the Necessity of Hospitals*

2.34   *Leverage the Voice of a Larger Organization to Accomplish Needed Change*

2.35   *Emerging Careers: Enhance the Training and Responsibility of the Apothecary*

2.36   *Meet a Community Need: Formation of the Cincinnati Eye Infirmary*

2.37   *Advocate for a School to Instruct the Blind*

2.38   *Competition as a Driver of Improvement*

2.39   *Indifference and Division among Members of a Community Hinder the Establishment of Institutions*

2.40   *Philanthropy Makes a Difference*

2.41   *Institutions Need Aspirational Goals to Guide Improvement*

Chapter Two

— *Establishing many residences in his lifetime, Drake was always devoted to improving his community and advocating on behalf of his fellow citizens. He created the first circulating library in Cincinnati in 1807, established the Kentucky School for the Blind in Louisville in 1830, and started the Cincinnati Medical Library Association in 1852.*

— *Drake was instrumental in constructing educational institutions that contributed to the vitality of education in Ohio and Kentucky. He began the School of Literature and Arts in 1813, and, most famously, he founded the Medical College of Ohio and Cincinnati College, which became part of the beginnings of the University of Cincinnati.*

— *He was a member of a number of societies related to his broad interests, including the Humane Society of Cincinnati, the Western Museum Society, the Cincinnati Society for the Promotion of Agriculture, Manufactures and Domestic Economy, and the Historical and Philosophical Society of Cincinnati.*

✠ AUTHOR INTRODUCTION

To leave a legacy as a citizen implies an individual has been engaged in solving the problems and addressing the needs of his or her community through selfless application of time, talent, and resources, and the person has left the community a better place as a result of those efforts. This brings to mind what Theodore Roosevelt proclaimed in his speech at the Sorbonne in Paris on April 23, 1910:

> It is not the critic who counts; not the man who points out how the strong man stumbles, or where the doer of deeds could have done them better. The credit belongs to the man who is actually in the arena, whose face is marred by dust and sweat and blood; who strives val-

> iantly; who errs, who comes short again and again, because there is no effort without error and shortcoming; but who does actually strive to do the deeds; who knows great enthusiasms, the great devotions; who spends himself in a worthy cause; who at the best knows in the end the triumph of high achievement, and who at the worst, if he fails, at least fails while daring greatly, so that his place shall never be with those cold and timid souls who neither know victory nor defeat.

This describes Daniel Drake's commitment to community life—never one to sit on the sidelines, he was devoted to worthy causes that mattered in a growing city.

The selections in this section show how Drake began by seeking to know his community's assets and people and also traveling to other cities and learning about their enduring institutions (2.1–2.13). He could see the need in a young city of growing a richer community culture through building the necessary infrastructure, and helping establish core and essential institutions such as libraries, schools, churches, museums, societies, hospitals, and specialty schools. He also advocated for systems for taking care of the poor and disabled (2.14–2.41). He applied his time as a leader and collaborator to establish a rich culture. His example illustrates how knowing people's needs and addressing those needs as a citizen changes the community for good. He promoted his community to the rest of the nation, and in so doing, attracted others to come and build there. As mentioned in the introduction, Sir William Osler, the great physician, said of Drake, "He started nearly everything in Cincinnati that is good and has lasted," and the truth of this statement endures.

2.1 Destiny Is Shaped by Where You Live

I expect from you a sort of intuitive acquiescence in the proposition, that the inhabitants of every country should be acquainted with its natural history. I anticipate from you an eager assent to the supplementary proposition, that a people in our situation have special need of an acquaintance with their productions and resources. With this conviction, which is equally the result of experience and reflection, you will be prepared to listen patiently to the feeblest exposition of the views and prospects of our society, so far as they involve the physical condition of the region in which our destinies are fixed.

An Anniversary Discourse, On the State and Prospects of the Western Museum Society. Cincinnati: Looker, Palmer, and Reynolds, 1820. 8.

READER REFLECTION

1. *What, in addition to the physical properties of a region, influences the destiny of the inhabitants (materially, in health or prosperity, in happiness)? Divide them into positive and negative factors.*
2. *What factors are working in your community? How can you change these factors for the good?*
3. *How does knowledge of the natural history of the region help alter the destiny of community?*

✖ 2.2 A REGION'S NATURAL ASSETS PREDICT ITS FUTURE

It will perhaps, to many persons at a distance, and particularly to those who have not studied our natural and commercial geography, appear altogether visionary, if not boastful, to speak of cities on these western waters. Yet it is certain, that those who have contemplated this country with most attention, are strongest in the belief, that many of the villages which have sprung up within 30 years, on the banks of the Ohio and Mississippi, are destined before the termination of the present century, to attain the rank of populous and magnificent cities. The grounds which support this prediction are too broad to be traveled over at this time; but it may be rendered plausible in a high degree, merely by a reference to the Mississippi. If we consider the quantity of water discharged by this great river—the vast extent and number of its branches, many of which exceed in length the largest rivers of Europe—the general direction of the main trunk, nearly from north to south, passing through more than 15° of latitude, in the temperate zone—the diversities of aspect, and inexhaustible fertility, of the region which it irrigates—the boundless and perennial forest, which in the east, and in the north, overshadowed its sources—the numerous beds of coal and iron which enrich its banks—the reciprocal ties and dependencies, which can never cease to operate, between the inhabitants of its upper and lower portions—numerous states which will possess in its navigation, a common interest, that must forever constitute a bond of political and commercial amity—we must be convinced that there is no river on earth of equal importance; or at least none on whose countless tributary streams so many millions can subsist.

Natural and Statistical View; or, Picture of Cincinnati and the Miami Country. Cincinnati: Looker and Wallace, 1815. 226, 227.

READER REFLECTION

1. *What are the current assets in your community that predicts your future? How can they be leveraged to secure the future?*
2. *Who needs to work together to use those assets most effectively?*

✸ 2.3 KNOW YOUR REGION'S TERRITORY

The map of the Miami country, which includes also the adjoining parts of Kentucky, so as to exhibit an entire view of the tracks depending on Cincinnati as their Emporium, has been compiled with much care by Mr. Thomas Danby, from the following materials, furnished him by the author: 1. The correct and beautiful map of Ohio, published in 1807, by the late captain JF Mansfield, from the official returns in the office of the surveyor general of the United States; 2. Transcripts from the plats in the office just mentioned, of such parts of this district as lie west of the state of Ohio; 3. A manuscript map of the counties watered by the Eastern branch of the Little Miami, procured from the auditor of the state; 4. A map of Campbell county, and Kentucky, furnished by General James Taylor, V.; and 5. Personal observation and research through most of the district, with oral and manuscript information from various persons.

Natural and Statistical View; or, Picture of Cincinnati and the Miami Country. Cincinnati: Looker and Wallace, 1815. viii–ix.

READER REFLECTION

1. *Part of knowing your community is defining its boundaries. How would you define your community to help map out the opportunities for improvement?*
2. *What resources would you employ (as Drake did) to define your community?*

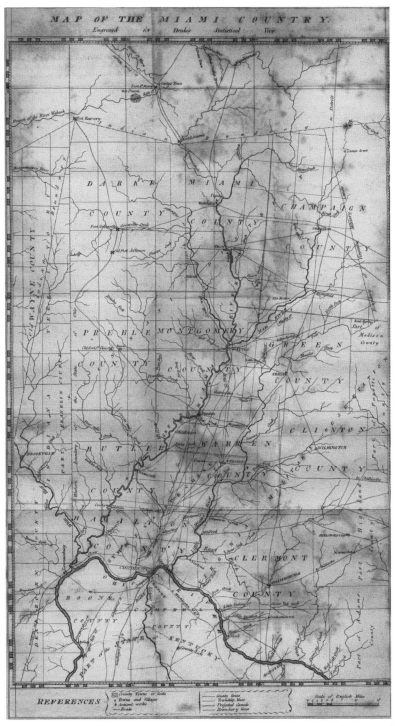

Map of the Miami Country included in Drake's 1815 book *Natural and Statistical View; or, Picture of Cincinnati and the Miami Country. Digital copy courtesy of the Henry R. Winkler Center for the History of Health Professions.*

✾ 2.4 Recognize the Value of Studying the Natural Resources of a Region

Our sandstone formation is extensive, and furnishes numerous quarries, whence building materials are conveyed to the towns and villages along our rivers. The strata of coal which it contains are of such extent, as to present an exhaustless supply of that important species of fuel, whenever the state of the country shall require them to be worked. Either this or the limestone formation, affords at least two valuable localities of Buhrstone [used to create millstones for grinding], sufficient, it is supposed, to supply the entire demand for that article, so important to an agricultural people. In both these formations there are many Salt springs, so strongly impregnated as to induce to the belief, that rock salt exists abundantly at no very great depth.

Our districts of slate are numerous; and from what has been discovered, there is no doubt that they contain beds of pyrites and aluminous shale, fit for the preparation of sulfur, sulfuric acid, alum, and copperas.

The alluvial formations of the Western Country, and especially of the states north of the Ohio, are extensive, and will doubtless yield their peculiar minerals in abundance. Those which are called wet prairies will probably afford peat and marl; the former of which may be regarded as indispensable to the growth of a dense population on tracts so destitute of wood. Beds of potter's clay are everywhere met within our alluvial grounds, and red and yellow ochres will doubtless be discovered. But the most important mineral supplied by these formations is iron, great quantities of which, in the state of our argillaceous oxide, unquestionably exist, and will be drawn from them by future industry.

Among the useful minerals which we may expect to find are mercury, zinc, antimony, and silver; the last of which in the state of sulphuret seems indeed have been already discovered.

An Anniversary Discourse, On the State and Prospects of the Western Museum Society. Cincinnati: Looker, Palmer, and Reynolds, 1820. 15, 16.

Reader Reflection

1. *What are/were the natural resources of the region where you live? How did those resources help shape your community? Have they changed or have they been exhausted? Or stewarded well?*

✖ 2.5 Record for Posterity How Your City Was Named: Cincinnati

In coming back in the month of January 1790 to Losantiville which we left with December 1789, we find it under a great nominal change; no longer designated by the original and auspicious epithet, which, composed of four tongues, gave presage of that variety in its people which the early future should contribute to its population; but known by the classical name which it now bears. An epitaph, equally dear to the lover of learning and the friend of freedom; recalling the purest days of Roman glory, and reminding us of the return by our revolutionary fathers from the field of blood to the field of peaceful industry. Till then it had never designated a city and even to this hour, it mysteriously remains, the cherished title of our beloved city only. When and by whom it was thus baptized will appear from the following extract of a letter from Judge [John C.] Symmes, which at the same time designates the author of the name by which our county has been known from the time of its organization.

"Governor [Arthur] St. Clair arrived at Losantiville on the second incident. He could be prevailed upon to stay with us but three nights. He has organized this purchase into a county—His Excellency complemented me with the honor naming the county—I called it Hamilton county after the secretary of the treasury [Alexander Hamilton]—General Harmer has named the new Garrison Fort Washington—the governor has made Losantiville the county town by the name of Cincinnati, so that Losantiville will become extinct.

Judge Luke Foster gives the following account of the colloquy on the subject. When governor St. Clair arrived from Fort Harmer, he came in a schooner. Israel Ludlow went on board, and the governor asked him what he called his town and was answered, "Losantiville."

"Give me," exclaimed the governor, "a name I can read and write!"
"Then, will you," said Ludlow, "please to name it?"
And St. Clair answered, "Let it be Cincinnati."

"Memoir of the Miami Country 1779–1794" [an unfinished manuscript for the Western Historical Society]. *Quarterly Publication of the Historical and Philosophical Society of Ohio* 18 (1923): 73–74.

Reader Reflection

1. How was your community named? Any meaning or story behind the name?

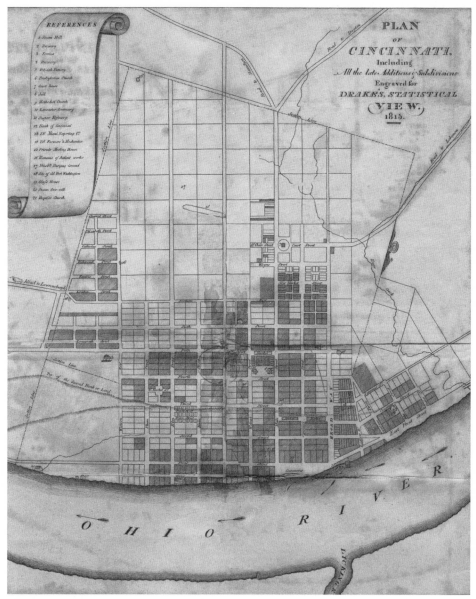

Map of the plan of the Cincinnati included in Drake's 1815 book *Natural and Statistical View; or, Picture of Cincinnati and the Miami Country. Digital copy courtesy of the Henry R. Winkler Center for the History of Health Professions.*

2.6 City Planning in Cincinnati

Philadelphia seems to have been the model after which that portion of this town first laid out, was planned. Between Broadway and Western Row there are six streets, each 66 feet wide, running from the River North 16° west, and lying 396 feet asunder. These are intersected at right angles by others of the same width, and at the same distance from each other; except Water and Front Street, and second and third Street, the former of which are nearer, and the latter, on account of the brow of the hill, more distant. Not a single alley, court, or diagonal street, and but one common, was laid out. The blocks or squares are each divided into eight lots, 99 by 198 feet, except those lying between second and third Street, which made 10 lots each; and those between front Water Street, the size of which may be seen by reference to the frontispiece. The out-lots, 81 in number, contain 4 acres each, and lie chiefly in the north of the town. The plan was not deposited in the public archives for record until 29 April, 1802. The streets in that part of the town laid out by John C. Symmes, are but 60 feet wide. Those intersecting the river run north 44° west, and lie at the same distance from each other as the streets in the original town; but the cross streets are nearer, and hence the lots of this quarter are shorter. The plan of this survey was not recorded by the proprietor until 12 September, 1811. The reservation of the general government was surveyed so as to connect the plots just described. The different subdivisions will be best understood by reference to the engraved plan.

Natural and Statistical View; or, Picture of Cincinnati and the Miami Country. Cincinnati: Looker and Wallace, 1815. 130–131.

READER REFLECTION

1. *How was your city planned or modeled? Does it still work for your community?*
2. *How has your community grown, and did this growth match the original plan?*
3. *What changes could be made to improve your current city plan?*

⊠ 2.7 PROMOTE THE ADVANTAGES OF YOUR COMMUNITY

Where will be erected the chief cities of this promising land? It may be answered with certainty—on the borders of the Ohio River. They are not likely to become places of political importance, for these must lie towards the centers of the states which this river will divide; but the commercial and manufactural advantages that exist in lieu of the political, are so much superior, as to justify, in this enqui-ry, the omission of every town not situated on the Ohio. Pittsburgh, Cincinnati, and Louisville are the places which at present have the fairest prospects of future greatness.... [T]here are reasons for believing that Cincinnati is to be the future metropolis of the Ohio. Its site is more eligible than that of most towns on the river. It is susceptible of being rendered healthier than Louisville, and is extensive enough for a large city. The Ohio bounds it on the south east, south, and south-west, so that all the streets, if extended, would at one or both ends intersect the river within the limits of the corporation. It has therefore a great extent of shore, along the whole of which there is not a reef nor shoal to prevent the landing of boats. Opposite to Broadway is the mouth of Licking; a river whose navigation will certainly be much improved. Over the town Plat,...a canal at some future period may be conducted from the great Miami; whose waters can, by another canal, be connected with those of the Maumee, and thus, secure to us a new and profitable trade with the lakes. A survey of the Ohio will exhibit us the important fact, that between Pittsburgh and Louisville there's not a single spot where a future rival to Cincinnati can be raised up. Finally, by reference to the map of the Miami country, it may be seen, that the river, in approaching Cincinnati from Maysville, which is 60 miles above, runs generally to the northwest; that after passing the town, it soon alters its course, and flows nearly to the south for more than 40 miles; and consequently, that Cincinnati lies in a situation to command the trade of the Eastern and Western, as well as interior portions of the Miami country. This is the case for more than 30 miles in those directions; and when the improvement of the roads shall be such as to facilitate intercourse of this place, the power it must exercise over these opposite districts will still be greater.

Natural and Statistical View; or, Picture of Cincinnati and the Miami Country. Cincinnati: Looker and Wallace, 1815.

Reader Reflection

1. *With knowledge of your area's natural resources, how can you promote the prospects and growth of your community?*
2. *Try envisioning what your community could become. What are the determinants of that vision?*

2.8 Know the Ethnic Groups in Your Community

The population of Cincinnati and its suburbs is 2320 souls. Of which number 1227 are males, 1013 are females, and 80 are Negros. The number of children under 16 years is 1051. The number of persons over 45 years is 184. The number who have attained the scriptural limit of the human life, three score and ten, is not known; but as men who have passed 60 years of age do not often immigrate to new and distant countries, instances in great longevity are not to be expected here. Indeed from the recent settlement of this place, few or none of its adult inhabitants are its natives. They have emigrated from every state in the union, and for most of the countries in the west of Europe; or especially Ireland, England, Germany, and Scotland. The American immigrants have been supplied principally by the states of north of Virginia.

A population derived from such distant sources, and so recently brought together, must necessarily exhibit much physical, as well as moral diversity. The climate and soil have not yet introduced a uniform constitutional body; nor customs, manners, and laws a uniform moral character. The inhabitants are generally laborious. By far the greatest number are mechanics. The rest are chiefly merchants, professional men, and teachers. Wealth is distributed more after the manner of the northern, than the southern states; and few or none are so independent, as to live without engaging in some kind of business.

Notices Concerning Cincinnati. Cincinnati: John W. Browne and Company, 1810. 30.

Reader Reflection

1. *The first step to help your community is to know the people who live there. Look around and see who lives in your community. How rich is the diversity? How is diversity defined in this time?*
2. *The United States is founded on immigration and developing a shared culture. What challenges are in your community in developing a shared culture inclusive of individuals of all races and ethnicities?*
3. *Is there such a thing as "moral character," and if so, how does the region in which we live impact the moral character of its citizens?*

2.9 Factors That Shift Community Demographics

The principal inducements for immigration to the State are, the fertility of its soil, the low prices of lands, an entire security of titles, the high price of labor, and the exclusion of slavery. For several years the Indian War opposed the operation of these inducements, but the Greenville treaty of 1795 brought them into full effect.

Fortunately, they happen to attract more attention, in the northern and middle states, which are at all times able to furnish the greatest number of immigrants. In the northern, especially, where the means of subsistence bear the smallest proportion to the population, these advantages have been fully appreciated, as it appears from the prevalence of the manners and customs of New England, over most of the state. The extraordinary emigration from that corner cannot be wholly contributed to these inducements, but has arisen in part from a portion of the north of the state being owned by Connecticut. In the same way the retention, by Virginia, of her right to the soil between the Little Miami and Scioto rivers, has been an additional motive with the people of that state for migrations to this. The prohibition of slavery has contributed greatly to the population of the state. The operation of this cause has not been confined to those states in which the practice of slavery is abolished, but has extended throughout the south, and is likely for many years to continue in full operation. It has even turned the current of European emigration from Kentucky and Tennessee, and spread it widely over Ohio.

Natural and Statistical View; or, Picture of Cincinnati and the Miami Country. Cincinnati: Looker and Wallace, 1815. 26, 27

READER REFLECTION

1. *What are the demographic changes taking place in your community?*
2. *What factors affect the demographic shifts in your community?*

⊞ 2.10 WHY OHIOANS ARE CALLED BUCKEYES

But why are the natives of our valley called Buckeyes?...

Every native of the valley of the Ohio should feel proud of the appellation, which, from the infancy of our settlements, has been conferred upon him; for the Buckeye has many qualities which may be typical of a noble character.

Beyond all the trees of the land, the Buckeye was associated with the family circle,—penetrating its privacy, facilitating its operations, and augmenting its enjoyments. Unlike many of its loftier associates, it did not bow its head and wave its arms at a haughty distance; but might be said to have held out the right hand of fellowship; for of all the trees of our forest, it is the only one with five leaflets arranged on one stem,—an expressive symbol of the human hand.

The Buckeye proved to be a friend indeed, because, in simple and expressive language of those early times, it was "a friend in need." Hats were manufactured of its fibers—the tray for delicious "pone" and "johnny-cake"—the venison trencher—the noggin—the spoon, and the huge white family bowl for mush and milk, were carved from its willing trunk.

In all our woods, there is not a tree so hard to kill as the Buckeye. The deepest girdling does not deaden it, and even after it is cut down and worked into the side of a cabin, it will send out young branches, denoting to all the world that Buckeyes are not easily conquered, and could with difficulty be destroyed.

The bark of the our emblem-plant has some striking properties—Under a proper method of preparation and use, it is said to be efficacious in the cure of malaria and fever, but unskillfully employed, it proves a violent emetic; which may indicate, that he who tampers with a Buckeye, will not do it with impunity.

The fruit of the Buckeye offers much to interest us. The capsule or covering of the nut is beset with sharp prickles, which, incautiously grasped, will soon compel the aggressor to let go his hold. The nut is undeniably the most beautiful of all which our teeming woods brings forth.... The inner covering of the nut is highly astringent. Its substance, when grated down, is soapy, and has been used to cleanse fine fabrics in the absence of good soap.

Who has not looked with admiration on the fine foliage of the Buckeye in early spring, while the more sluggish tenants of the forest remain torpid in their winter quarter; and what tree in all our wild woods, bears a flower which can be compared with that of our favorite....

My object has been to show the peculiar fitness of the Buckeye to be made the symbol-tree of our native population. This arises from its many excellent qualities. Other trees may have greater magnitude, and stronger trunks. They are the Hercules of the forest; and like him of old, who was distinguished only for physical power, they are remarkable chiefly for their mechanical strength. Far different it is with the Buckeye, which does not depend on brute force to effect its objects; but exercises, as it were, a moral power, and admonishes all who adopt its name, to rely upon intellectual cultivation, instead of bodily prowess.

"The Description of the Buckeye." [Excerpted from an address given by Daniel Drake at a dinner to celebrate the forty-fifth anniversary of the first settlement of Cincinnati, December 26, 1833.] In *The Akron Offering: A Ladies' Literary Magazine, 1849–1850*, edited by Jon Miller. Akron, OH: University of Akron Press Publications, 2013. 160–167.

General William Henry Harrison also attended this dinner, and it was during his 1840 election campaign seven years later that the term Buckeyes referring to Ohioans was popularized with commemorative walking sticks part of the campaign memorabilia.

1. *What symbol, based on the specific qualities of that symbol, would you choose for your family or company?*

2.11 ENVISION AN ENDURING COMMUNITY CULTURE

Thus, connected by nature in the great Valley, you must live in the bonds of companionship, or imbrue our lands in each other's blood. We have no middle destiny. To secure the former to our posterity, we should begin while society is still tender and pliable. The saplings of the woods, if intertwined, will adapt themselves to each other and grow together; the little bird may hang its nest on the twins of different trees, and the dew-drop fall successively on leaves which are nourished by distinct trunks. The tornado strikes harmless on such a tree bow, for the various parts sustain each other; but the growing tree; sturdy and set in its way; will not bend to its fellow, and when uprooted by the tempest, is dashed in violence against all within his reach.

Communities, like forest, go rigid by time. They properly trained must be molded while young. Our duty, then, is quite obvious. All who have moral power, should exert it in concert. The germs of harmony must be nourished, and the roots of present contrariety or future discord torn up and cast into the fire. Measures should be taken to mold a uniform system of manners and customs, out of the diversified elements which are scattered over the west. Literary meetings should be held in the different states; and occasional conventions in the central cities of the great Valley, be made to bring into friendly consultation, our enlightened and zealous teachers, professors, lawyers, physicians, the divines, and men of letters, from its remotest sections. In their deliberations the literary and moral wants of the various regions might be made known, and the means of supplying them devised. The whole should successively lend a helping hand to all the parts, on the great subject of education from the primary school to the university. Statistical facts, bearing on this absorbing interest, should be brought forward and collected; the systems of common school instruction should be compared, and the merits of different schoolbooks, foreign and domestic, freely canvassed. Plans of education, adapted to the natural, commercial, and social condition of the interior, should be invented; a correspondence instituted among all our higher seminaries of learning, and an interchange established of all local publications on the subject of education. In short, we should foster western genius, encourage western writers, patronize western publishers, augment the number of western readers, and create a western heart.

When these great objects shall come seriously to occupy our minds, the union will be secure, for its center will be sound, and its attraction on the surrounding parts irresistible. Then will our state governments emulate each other in works for the common good; the people of remote places begin to feel as the members of one family; and our whole intelligent and virtuous population unite, heart and hand in one long, concentrated, untiring effort, to raise still higher the social character, and perpetuate forever, the political harmony of the green and growing West.

"Remarks on the Importance of Promoting Literary and Social Concert, in the Valley of the Mississippi, as a Means of Elevating Its Character and Perpetuating the Union." [Delivered at the Literary Convention of Kentucky, November 8, 1833, in the chapel of Transylvania University.] Louisville: Members of the Convention at the Office of the *Louisville Herald*, 1833. 25–26.

READER REFLECTION

Drake recognized the emerging western states were made up of immigrants from many different countries and was more diverse than the original thirteen colonies. He saw this as an asset, but what was needed were a common culture. One of the ways to do this was through education and social institutions made up of moral individuals with literary interests. He foresaw that these were means to preserve and strengthen the union of states.

1. *What happens when a society fails to recognize the value inherent in diverse people coming together with the goal of forming an enduring community?*
2. *Catalog the types of culture-building gatherings in your community. Do they include any of those listed by Drake in this selection? Do they work to build a common culture or keep groups separate?*

✖ 2.12 REWARD AND PUNISHMENT GOVERN HUMAN BEHAVIOR AND ARE THE FOUNDATION OF SOCIETY

Was there but one man, it would be necessary to his welfare that he should not violate the laws, which regulate the relations between him and the surrounding elements; for if he did, he would suffer bodily pain, and perhaps perish. Thus, if he exposed himself, unprotected, to the north wind, at midnight in winter, he would be frozen; or, if he walked into the fire, he would be burnt—in both cases, receiving the penalty imposed on the violation; while on the other hand, if he scrupulously observed the laws which regulate the relations between his system and heat and cold, his feelings would be pleasant, and, in that pleasure, he would find the reward of his fidelity to the requirements of his physical nature.

Again, if we contemplate him associated with others in society, and suppose him to violate the laws which are necessary to its government and well being, we see him doomed to suffer a penalty; while on the contrary, a strict observance of all the regulations of social compact never fails to preserve his peace, and procure for him the reward of conscious rectitude, and the approbation and confidence of his fellow. Thus, both in the world of matter and the world of mind, we find punishment the consequence of violation, and reward the beneficial effect of obedience.

When we come to inquire into the reason of this relation between the act and its consequence, we at once perceive that without it, no law would be respected; and that, in the economy of the world, rewards and punishments are appointed means of securing obedience, and maintaining the supremacy of those enactments, domestic, social, political, and moral, without which men could not live in each other's society.

"Discipline: Discourse on the Philosophy of Family, School, and College Discipline." *Transactions of the Fourth Annual Meeting of the Western Literary Institute and College of Professional Teachers.* [Meeting held in Cincinnati, October 1834.] Cincinnati: Josiah Drake Publisher, 1835. 32–33.

READER REFLECTION

1. *Long before psychology as a field was created, Drake recognized that behavior has consequences and reward and punishment are fundamental motivators of human behavior. Are there current behaviors for which the rewards or consequences appear to be, or have become, ineffective?*

2. *In your community are there clear rewards for promoting social harmony and effective deterrents for negative behaviors?*

✠ 2.13 A Universal Principle Providing Safety and Undergirding a Free Society

The last principle of action to which I shall direct your inquiries, is veneration for God. This, like the others, is innate, and the highest of all moral sentiments....

Veneration, in its perfect degree, involves gratitude, love, and respect; but the two former are not indispensable, for we often cherish the latter alone. Indeed, respect is but a lower degree of veneration, and this is what we feel for a great and good name of antiquity, or an ancient and beneficial custom. Reverence is the same feeling, cherished for things that are divine, or for persons who seem to stand as representatives of the divinity, such as pious or aged parents, or exemplary and hoary-headed teachers, or ministers of the gospel.

The veneration or reverence of children for their parents, and preceptors, should comprehend love and gratitude and respect, and be ennobled with a looking up to God, as the fountain of whatever is lovely and reverential in them. Thus formed and directed, this sentiment gives to the parent and teacher, a control over the will and actions of the child, beyond every other.... When this feeling is exists, the fear of incurring the displeasure of the parent or preceptor, is constantly present, and constitutes a powerful means of prevention, while it keeps down anger and resentment under correction, if that be necessary. The setting up of the authority of this sentiment of adoration to God and reverence for the parent, in the heart of a child, is the great desideratum in discipline, from the cradle to the theatre of life—from the primary school, to the university. It is an aegis of brass against immorality, and the palladium of liberty, in every land where freedom is sustained by a constitutional government. The power of this principle, in a national point of view, is disclosed, by the hesitation with which the subjects of a throne, held venerable by tradition and early impressions, come up to is overthrow; although it may have sent forth none but the edicts of despotism. The heroes of the revolution, and the authors of the federal constitution and union it establishes, should be held up to our children, as patriots whom they ought to reverence—the works themselves as political institutions which deserve the deepest veneration. This should be part of their education, at home, in society, in the primary school, the academy, and the university; for a great object of education in this country is to make good citizens, and devoted friends of liberty we now enjoy. The spread of this feeling of reverence throughout the whole republic would in no degree interfere with all necessary amendments to the constitution, but rather contribute to promote them, while it would affords the greatest of all possible guarantees against its abolition, by combinations of wicked men, in whom the sentiment of reverence for what is good never finds a place....

Children who are taught to venerate their parents and teachers; the fathers of the land who have labored for its prosperity; our aged and virtuous matrons; our benevolent, literary, and religious institutions; and those who conduct them on correct principles—finally, Heaven itself, for which they all labor, become a law unto themselves, and conform, in manhood, to what they venerated in youth.

Reverence for God, as a first and great unseen, governing power, is a universal principle of human nature, which in different ages and nations, has made itself manifest in various ways, according to the lights of understanding. Thus among the ancients, while the Egyptians bowed down in blind adoration to the filthiest reptiles, the Greeks paid homage to the creations of a bright but licentious imagination; and in one of the kingdoms of modern Europe [France], when delivered over to a civil war and drenched with innocent blood, though philosophy raised her voice above the din of anarchy, and proclaimed there is no God, the people erected alters to the worship of Nature! The sentiment of devotion may be sunk, obscured and perverted, but cannot be abolished.... They who are instructed in the Bible view the Creator as the author of rewards as well as punishments, and love him with gratitude while they fear him in humility. They know his attributes and decrees, and humble themselves before him as a being of infinite wisdom and goodness—worthy of all veneration—whose revealed will commands every moral duty—whose law of universal kindness—who enjoins justice and generosity.

"Discipline: Discourse on the Philosophy of Family, School, and College Discipline." *Transactions of the Fourth Annual Meeting of the Western Literary Institute and College of Professional Teachers.* [Meeting held in Cincinnati, October 1834.] Cincinnati: Josiah Drake Publisher, 1835. 57–59.

READER REFLECTION

1. *Discuss: "Reverence for God...is a universal principle of human nature."*
2. *What does Drake say is the consequence of revering God (and, by extension, one's parents) on human society?*

⊠ 2.14 Take Care of the Poor

No pauper is by law entitled to support from the township, without the residence of one year. The common mode of maintaining those who are permanent charges is to offer them annually to the lowest bidder. The funds for defraying this expense, and for the support of poor generally, are raised by an annual tax on the same species of property which is taxed for county purposes.

With the design of extending charity to the needy, who in consequence of their recent arrival here can demand nothing from the overseers of the poor; and to those citizens who are, through misfortune, and in want of temporary assistance, a number of charitable persons associated themselves in 1814, under the name of the Cincinnati Benevolent Society. They appointed two managers in each ward of the town, and by the voluntary contribution of a respectable portion of the inhabitants, a sum was obtained that has enabled the society to dispense relief to a number of suffering immigrants. A part of the design, which will perhaps be here after executed, is the erection of the work house; where those who are unable entirely to support themselves, or find assistance, and be compelled to labor according to their abilities. Another important establishment by this society, would be a dispensary, for the relief in sickness, of those families who in the health do not require gratuitous assistance.

Natural and Statistical View; or, Picture of Cincinnati and the Miami Country. Cincinnati: Looker and Wallace, 1815. 173.

Reader Reflection

1. *What social services exist for the poor in your community? Do those services require some sort of work according to the person's ability? Discuss how to do this in a just and compassionate manner.*
2. *What health care services exist for the poor in your community? What are the challenges facing those services?*

⊠ 2.15 Call Out the Consequences of a Bad Law—The Fugitive Slave Act of 1850

Fugitism is a great and growing national calamity. The increase of Negroes in the North, and of intelligence among the free Negroes and slaves of the South; with the multiplication of steamboats, and the construction of railroads, the means of escape will increase, and fugitism enlarge its borders: the General Government has no right to interfere, nor power to prevent it, if the right existed. That government can only assist a master in reclaiming his slave; but reclamation is not prevention. The present fugitive law will be sustained. Its repeal will dissolve the Union at once; but its execution will certainly lead to the same sad catastrophe at no very distant day. Every case of arrest will continue to be of new source of irritation in the North: every unsuccessful trial, an equal source of anger and resentment in the South. He who visits the former to reclaim a slave will return with curses on his lips, to be followed with the curses of those among whom he had adventured. It requires no spirit of prophecy to foresee the disastrous result of such crimination between political brethren; nor any deep-toned patriotism to pray for its early extinction. [Letter Two]

"Letters on Slavery to John C. Warren of Boston." The *National Intelligencer* [Washington, DC], April 3, 5, and 7, 1851.

Reader Reflection

The Fugitive Slave Law was passed on September 18, 1850, as part of the 1850 Compromise between the slave-holding South and the free North. Only six months after the law had passed Drake observed some of the early consequences and predicted that it was highly likely that the Union would be dissolved (civil war).

1. *Are there any laws currently being debated on the state or national level that will have negative consequences on the social order?*
2. *What can you do to influence the debate in a positive way?*

2.16 Love Is Needed to Address Social Disparities

Christianity cannot take the heart by human violence. The soul of Christianity is love; the fruit of Christianity is love. This love binds heart to heart, inspires mutual confidence, and makes men who dwell together in the same house of one mind. When master and slave are brought under its influence, they become spiritual brethren; one is humbled, the other exalted. In all that relates to a common eternity, they live and move on the same platform; and we forget all we ever learned of human nature when we affirm that such an equality will not cause the master to regard with deeper interest the temporal wants of the slaves—his brothers in Christ. Let us, then, I repeat, place reliance on this Divine Influence; let us wait with patience the progress of that moral and social reformation which has already soothed the sorrows of so many slaves; let us abide the appointed time, and look with hope to the Christian spirit of the age for all that can be done to hasten the great work of emancipation. [Letter One]

This natural inferiority to the white man has been given as a reason for reducing [the slave] to bondage. But the heartlessness of such an argument is only equaled by its logical absurdity; for where there is a disparity, in mental and moral power, the legitimate conclusion is that the stronger should help, not prey, upon the weaker. To reverse this is to set aside the laws of the moral world, and establish a reign of force and anarchy. [Letter Two]

"Letters on Slavery to John C. Warren of Boston." The *National Intelligencer* [Washington, DC], April 3, 5, and 7, 1851.

READER REFLECTION

In the spirit of the times, Drake believed that "God created varieties of men, some which are superior to others." He also recognized that slaves with "aspirations after equality will become inflamed," and, "aided by" whites, will "attempt by force to acquire greater privileges or seek revenge for what is withheld from them. Thus rebellions, amounting to local civil wars, will carry dismay throughout our cities, and drench our streets with blood." He recognized the current social order in the United States including the North, "forever chilled and palsied the aspirations of Negroes." As a consequence he promoted a solution to create a free colony in Africa where "his [the Negro's] energies of mind and of body might have ample scope," and "where the wings of ambition" may have an "open atmosphere of perfect liberty and independence" [Letter Two].

1. *Does your community have explicit or implicit social structures that perpetuate disparities? Seek to identify those that exist and ask what needs to be done.*

2. *Are there opportunities to help those who are "weaker" or are there examples of groups of people who are taken advantage of by others even implicitly? By what principles do you believe that individuals should help the "weaker"? The same as Drake espoused?*

3. *How can love for all in your community be practically introduced?*

⊠ 2.17 Recognize the Social Forces Driving Behaviors in the Community

Fashion is rooted in that principle of human nature, which makes "man an imitative animal"; and involves that sentiment, which leads him to respect public opinion. Few persons, therefore, are raised above the influence of fashion, and that few, are none the better for their forced and unsocial elevation. It is one thing, however, to set fashion at defiance; another to become its victim. Fashion, to a greater or less extent, is the taste and opinions of the world embodied. It is therefore always entitled to attention, if not to respect. It is characteristic of good sense and sound principal, to examine into the requirements of fashion, and conform to them, as far as the accord with nature, propriety and convenience. It is the vain and frivolous, only, that yields a blind submission. Good taste rejects all that is absurd or ridiculous: bad taste swallows the whole without examination. Fashion exerts the greatest domination over young minds; and in youth, acts upon both sexes in nearly the same degree. Education being equal, the weakest minded are the greatest devotees of fashion; but in early life it imparts delight to every grade of intellect, though in varying degrees. Young persons, are not aware of the delusions of fashion, should be admonished, against yielding to its absurd demands. I do not know a harder master. It has no heart, no conscience, no stability. It governs without law, and sentences without a hearing. It changes, like epidemic diseases, come and go, when we least expect them; and often with the social devastation which might carry out the metaphor. No perspicacity can foresee its caprices, or prepare to meet them. The edicts of the morning are reversed before the evening lamp of pleasure and dissipation is extinguished. That which it lauds today, it scorns tomorrow, and ridicules those who joined in the praise. Such is its character.

An Oration on the Causes, Evils, and Preventives of Intemperance. Columbus: Olmstead & Bailhache, Printers, 1831. 9, 10.

Reader Reflection

1. *People are social animals and influenced by the latest trends or fads. What trends or fads are happening in your community or field of work that are capturing the attention of most? What are the positive or negative impacts of these?*
2. *How strongly influenced are you by the opinions and thoughts of others?*

✠ 2.18 THE VALUE OF A MUSEUM DISPLAYING THE GREAT CIRCLE OF KNOWLEDGE

As the arts and sciences have not hitherto been cultivated among us to any great extent, the influence they are capable of exerting on our happiness and dignity is not generally perceived, and they have consequently but few friends and admirers. It is therefore proper, that we should institute and continue to observe an annual festival in celebration of the origin of a society established expressly for their promotion; that we may elevate their character with a mass of our people, and multiply the number of their devotees and patrons, by the infallible method of augmenting their consequence.

The plan of our establishment embraces nearly the whole of those parts of the great circle of knowledge, which require material objects, either natural or artificial, for their illustration. It has, of course, a variety of subdivisions, and in its execution will call for very different architects, as its consummation will afford instruction and delight to persons of many opposite taste. Already, indeed, in possession of many specimens in Zoology, Mineralogy, Antiquities, and the Fine and Useful Arts, we venture to indulge the hope, that even at this time, we can offer something to interested naturalist, antiquary and the mechanician.

An Anniversary Discourse, On the State and Prospects of the Western Museum Society. Cincinnati: Looker, Palmer, and Reynolds, 1820. 5, 6.

READER REFLECTION

1. *What is the value of museums to a community? Consider supporting a museum of your choice, or consider a trip to a local museum to learn about the collection and add to your own knowledge.*
2. *How can one publicize the value of such institutions to the community?*

✠ 2.19 HOW A COLLEGE AND A MUSEUM COMPLEMENT ONE ANOTHER

These reflections naturally suggest the propriety of adverting to the introduction of the museum into the College edifice where we are now assembled [Chapel of the Cincinnati College]. This connection will, in all probability, be made permanent, and may be regarded as auspicious for both institutions. In some degree they are necessary to the success of one another, and the interest of both would, therefore, suffer by a separation. They afford, in succession, all the aids that are essential to a liberal education. The College is principally a school of literature, the Museum of science and the arts. The knowledge imparted by one is elementary, by the other practical. Without the former, our sons would be illiterate; without the latter, they would be scholars merely—by the help of both, they may become scholars and philosophers.

An Anniversary Discourse, On the State and Prospects of the Western Museum Society. Cincinnati: Looker, Palmer, and Reynolds, 1820. 26, 27.

READER REFLECTION

1. *Your community has many institutions. Which institutions complement and assist each other? Is there opportunity to for them to work together to strengthen their missions and their value to the community?*

✠ 2.20 STUDY AND MEMORIALIZE THE PAST IN YOUR COMMUNITY

Our country exhibits older and nobler monuments than the recent vestiges of our Indian tribes. The number, extent, and regularity of our mounds, and the implements of stone and copper which they contain, afford incontestable proofs that a people more numerous, enlightened, and thoughtful, than the wandering hordes found on the discovery of the continent had previously been its inhabitants. These monuments are our only antiquities; and although they may not, like the classical ruins of Asia and Europe, awaken inspiration, nor infuse melancholy, they will not, I hope, be thought altogether unworthy of our admiration. At what time where they erected, and deserted; have the people who formed them become extinct; did they immigrate to Mexico; or slowly degenerate into the existing hordes, and what were the causes of any of these events, are problems which can be solved only by researches into the relics which they have left. These should be vigilantly sought after and carefully preserved, that they may be compared with each other and works of art which belong to the existing tribes. We should thus snatch from the grave a memorial of the former condition of our country, and gain at least a few materials for the portrait of a people, whose very name is blotted from the tablet of humanity.

An Anniversary Discourse, On the State and Prospects of the Western Museum Society. Cincinnati: Looker, Palmer, and Reynolds, 1820. 20, 21.

1. *Communities have a story of origin. How well memorialized are the people who came before you? Is there an opportunity to create a story of the past to bring people together in a spirit of unity and pride?*

2. *Are there biases in the way we view the past, and if so, what are these biases, and how can we capture them as teaching points while rectifying them and not lose our community's story?*

⊠ 2.21 APPRECIATE, SUPPORT, AND PROMOTE THE FINE ARTS

I have already announced, that the promotion of the useful and ornamental arts, is among the objects of our society. Drawings, models, and products of the former, whether a mechanical or chemical, will find a conspicuous place; and every exertion will be made to acquire good specimens of the latter. Having been transplanted from countries where the fine arts were flourishing in vigor and beauty, our people, in general, are not without the relish for them. Those, indeed, who have once gazed with admiration on the sublime historical combinations of a West, or the faithful portraits of individual greatness by a Stewart, can never lose the taste for that enjoyment. Should any person object to the gratification of this taste, as a luxury that ought to be prohibited in the young republic, I would reply, that the cultivation of the fine arts should be regarded merely as a concomitant and not as the cause, for the consequence, of a luxurious state of society, and that a love for the chaste and elegant labors of the painter, the architect, and the sculptor, should not be ranked with the relish for the pleasures of the table, an admiration for personal ornaments, and a passion for public shows, and dissolute amusements. The former originates in sentiment, and its gratification imparts dignity and elevation, the latter are rooted in sensuality, vanity and vice, and their indulgence leads to ruin and disgrace.

> One springs from "faculties that walk the range of heaven,"
> The others from "appetites that grovel on the earth."

It may be said, however, that we are too poor to encourage the fine arts. I will admit that but a few of our citizens have sufficient wealth to become their individual patrons, but this very circumstance constitutes a strong argument for confiding to a collective body, the means and the duty of promoting their introduction into this country. This object has been assigned to our society, and I hope to see it executed in a manner that will both delight and refine the public taste.

An Anniversary Discourse, On the State and Prospects of the Western Museum Society. Cincinnati: Looker, Palmer, and Reynolds, 1820. 23–24.

Reader Reflection

1. *Are the fine arts valued by the general public in your community? What does it compete with for time and support? Who are the patrons?*
2. *How can you assist with supporting the fine arts?*

2.22 Create a Lecture Series for the Public Good

Among the variety of objects which it is designed to embrace in the museum, are several kinds of philosophical instruments, calculated to illustrate the principles of magnetism, electricity, galvanism, mechanics, hydrostatics, optics, and the mechanism of the solar system. The whole of these can be fabricated by an ingenious curator, Mr. Best, and the acquisition of them will not only facilitate the progress of the solitary student, but enable the society to institute public lectures on the different branches of natural philosophy, as well as of zoology, mineralogy, geology, American antiquities, and the fine arts. Popular courses on the subject, delivered from time to time, as the means of illustration become adequate, and competent lecturers can be engaged, would accord with the spirit that suggested the establishment of the museum, and could not fail to multiply the benefits which it is expected to confer.

An Anniversary Discourse, On the State and Prospects of the Western Museum Society. Cincinnati: Looker, Palmer, and Reynolds, 1820. 24, 25.

Reader Reflection

1. *Here is an example of creating a forum for public lectures for the benefit of the community. Does your community have such opportunities? Would there be a lecture that you could give or one you would enjoy hearing?*

✄ 2.23 Promote the Value of Books

One of the most painful deprivations experienced by the student of nature in these new and remote settlements, is the want of books to direct his researches.... Without their assistance, indeed, we can neither comprehend nor enjoy the wider and brighter prospects, which our superior elevation of affords, but most resemble navigators becalmed in sight of new lands, abounding in all that could reward them for the perils and privations of the voyage; or guests bidden to a feast, and when seated, prohibited from tasting the luxuries which tantalize their longing appetites. We may be encompassed by a thousand interesting objects—our feet may press the rarest productions of the mineral world, and on every side the most beautiful forms of living nature may smile upon us and invite our scrutiny, but the whole will be unavailing. It is not given to us, to penetrate by a single glance, the veil which the Creator has thrown over the relations, that bind it into one beautiful and admirable system, the myriad of parts which compose the mighty fabric of this globe.

Thousands of years have elapsed since the students of nature begin to unfold her mysteries. Books are the great repository of their discoveries, and he who neglects them, begins, like the first observer, unaided and alone. He may be compared to the astronomer who, rejecting the records of the science, and even refusing to employ the telescope, might continue at the base of the observatory, and contemplate the heavens with the unassisted vision. Surrounded then, as we are by a multitude of curious and important productions, we cannot, I think, refrain from introducing and consulting the oracles which might aid us in assigning their names in acquiring a knowledge of the history and qualities.

An Anniversary Discourse, On the State and Prospects of the Western Museum Society. Cincinnati: Looker, Palmer, and Reynolds, 1820. 25, 26.

Reader Reflection

1. *Drake was an example of a person who was largely self-taught, and books allowed him to advance quickly to a broader understanding of life. He helped found a public library and then also Medical Library for Cincinnati. Are you a user and possibly a patron of your local library?*

2. *How did you become a reader? Do you have a reading program that allows you to move beyond a "first observer, unaided and alone"—and have your "vision assisted"?*

✠ 2.24 CREATE A LITERARY SOCIETY

Our first year's labors were closed, by the interesting discourse, which has just been read. During that period, we have assembled, for literary exercise, more than 20 times.... The objects and character of our infant association have been defined and established; an impetus has been given it, and regular exertion only is wanting, to raise it into notice and respectability.

The essays of the members, if less learned and profound, have equaled all reasonable expectation. Some of them consist chiefly of original matter, while others manifest the degree of research, which is honorable to their authors, and auspicious to the school.

It would be amusing to review the contents but being restricted to limits too narrow for that undertaking, I will substitute a catalog of their titles:

1. an essay on education
2. on the earthquakes of 1811, 1812, and 1813
3. on light
4. on carbon
5. on air
6. on the mind
7. on agriculture
8. on caloric
9. on gravitation
10. on instinct
11. notices of the aurora borealis of 17 April and 11 September 1814
12. an essay on water, considered chemically and hydrostatically
13. on common sense
14. on heat
15. on the mechanical powers
16. on the theory of earthquakes
17. on enthusiasm
18. on the geology of Cincinnati and its personality illustrated with mineral specimens in a vertical map
19. on the internal commerce of the United States
20. on hydrogen
21. on rural economy
22. on the geology of some parts of New York and
23. on general commerce

Such, briefly, is the character of our introductory labors. Their retrospection cannot fail to excite a portion of complacency and hope in ourselves, though from my fellow citizens they may extort neither the need of approbation nor the humble reward of occasional attendance. These, however, are certainly attainable. Our lot, gentlemen, is cast in a region abundant in but a few things, except the products of a rich and unexhausted soil. Learning, philosophy, and taste are yet in early infancy, and the standard of excellence in literature and science is proportionately low. Hence, acquirements, which older and more enlightened countries would scarcely raise an individual to mediocrity, will here place him in a commanding station. Those who attain superiority in the community in which they are members are relatively great. Literary excellence in Paris, London, or Edinburgh is incomparable with the same thing in Philadelphia, New York, or Boston: while each of these, in turn, has a standard of merit, which may be contrasted, but not compared, with that of Lexington or Cincinnati. Still, comparative superiority in Europe, the Atlantic states or Back-woods, is equally gratifying; and gives to him who possesses it, the same influence over the community to which he belongs.

But it will, perhaps, be assertive, that in a state so young as this, no literary distinction is attainable, that would out value its cost; that academies and colleges are as yet scarcely instituted; that libraries, philosophical apparatus, and scientific teachers are equally rare and imperfect; that associations for improvement, animated and impelled by a persevering spirit, can find a habitation in these rude and checkered settlements; and, lastly, that our countrymen are accustomed to look with frigid in difference on every species of literary effort. This is, indeed, pouring cold water on the flame of literary ambition: but that noble passion is not to be thus extinguished; and if a single spark remain, it will enable us to proceed, through the Gothic darkness which envelopes our literature and science, the certain though narrow paths to a brighter region.

Anniversary Address, Delivered to the School of Literature and the Arts at Cincinnati, November 23, 1814. Cincinnati: Looker and Wallace, 1814. 3–5.

READER REFLECTION

1. *Do you belong to a group of individuals who are interested in preparing papers on and discussing the great questions of the day? What benefit is gained from such groups or organizations? In knowledge and building community?*
2. *How do you persevere in the face of general indifference?*

✖ 2.25 THE CRITICAL ROLE OF ROADS FOR ENHANCING COMMERCE

The project of constructing, between the Miamies, from Cincinnati towards the source of these rivers, a great road, which should at all seasons be equally passable, has been for sometime in agitation. It will perhaps be undertaken in 1816, and pass by the nearest route from this town to Dayton. The benefits which an execution of this plan would confer, cannot be fully estimated, except by those who have traveled to the Miami country in the winter season, and have studied the connections in business between that district and Cincinnati. The salt, the iron, the castings, the glass, the cotton, and the foreign merchandise for at least eight counties will be transported on this road; which would immediately become one of the most important in the state.

Natural and Statistical View; or, Picture of Cincinnati and the Miami Country. Cincinnati: Looker and Wallace, 1815. 220.

READER REFLECTION

1. Reliable roads are essential for building community cohesiveness and the local economy. Does your community have the capacity for what is needed? Are systems of transportation optimized? What improvements or innovations are needed?

✖ 2.26 RECOMMENDED IMPROVEMENTS TO FACILITATE COMMUNITY CONNECTIONS

Under this head I do not propose to mention any other improvements than those which are calculated to facilitate the intercourse between the town and country....

Canals. To discharge a portion of the waters of the Great Miami into the Ohio, at this town, would, confessedly, be a great public benefit; but no proposition on this subject has yet appeared; nor does it seem to have attracted much attention. In the whole course of the Miami, there is perhaps but one point where a canal could be opened; and that is near Hamilton, 25 miles from the mouth of the river, and about the same distance from Cincinnati. In the valley, five miles south of the former town, there is a large pond, which is replenished by the Miami, when that river is high; and out of which, at the same time, arises one of the principal branches of Mill-creek. From this place to Cincinnati, following the meanders of the stream, there is nothing to prevent the opening of a canal. The valley, it is true, contains great quantities of pebbles and gravel covered with soil, but by keeping near the hills that bound it, an argillaceous [fine, clay sediment] bottom could be had. The difference in level, at low water, between the Ohio at this town, and the Miami at Hamilton, has not been ascertained; but it may be estimated at 60 feet. About four miles from Cincinnati, the canal would have to be carried over Mill-creek, after which it might be conducted along the base of the high lands which border the site of the town on the north, to the valley of Deer-creek, through which it would reach the Ohio.

The time when the enterprise and resources of the citizens of the Miami country will be adequate to the execution of this project, cannot be foretold; but when we consider the ratio of our progression in strength and numbers within the last fifteen years, there is much reason to hope that the era of this improvement is not remote. The transportation on this canal and the Miami above (if its navigation were somewhat improved) would, in less than half a century, be great indeed. The country on each side, for the average distance of 25 miles, and as far north as the navigable waters of the Maumee, about 110, would be dependent on it. In this parallelogram of 5500 square miles, there is no spot which is not susceptible of cultivation; and by far the greater part is equal to any land in the United States. It only, therefore, requires facilities for the exportation of its surplus produce, and the importation of foreign articles, to ensure for it a very dense population; and such facilities would be afforded by the canal. In addition to this, should the difficulties connected with the navigation of the Maumee and its branches be removed at the same time, the skins and peltry, the fish, and perhaps the copper of the north, would reach the Ohio; and the cotton, sugar, tobacco, and other productions of the south would pass into the Lakes through the same channel.

[Construction of the Miami and Erie Canal (274 miles) that ran from Toledo, OH, began in 1825 and was finished in 1845. Commercial use ended in 1913.]

Natural and Statistical View; or, Picture of Cincinnati and the Miami Country. Cincinnati: Looker and Wallace, 1815. 224–225.

READER REFLECTION

1. *One of the fundamentals for improving, growing, and building a community is assessing the resources and then encouraging and creating ways to build and exchange those assets. What assets do you have in your community? Are there ways yet to be developed that would open up those assets to more individuals?*

2. *Sometimes exchanges are limited by physical barriers yet to be overcome; other times they can be social barriers to be overcome. What barriers limit the exchange of assets in your community and to other communities?*

2.27 Proposing and Predicting the Benefits of a Railroad from Cincinnati to Charleston

The states which border on the Ohio, or are watered by its great tributary streams, are western or tramontane Pennsylvania and Virginia, Ohio, Indiana, Illinois, Kentucky, and Tennessee; nearly through the center of which that river flows, almost parallel with the sea coast of the old southern states. From the seven states above mentioned, there are highways of communication from the ocean in two directions—northeast and southwest. The former, consisting of several distinct lines of river, canal, macadamized, and railroad communication, reaches the Atlantic ocean between the west end of Long Island Sound and the mouth of the Chesapeake Bay from New York to Norfolk—a distance, on a straight line, of 300 miles: the latter communicates with the Gulf of Mexico by the delta of the Mississippi. Between these two points of marine connection with the interior is a coast nearly 3000 miles in extent, constituting the sea-board of southern Virginia, North and South Carolina, Georgia, Florida, Alabama, and Mississippi, with which the states in the Valley of the Ohio have no direct communication, even by means of a good post-road, so that the mail to the northern frontier of Georgia and the Carolinas, not three hundred miles distant from the banks of the Ohio, in a straight line, is actually sent by Washington City, on a route nearly four times as long. With that part of the southern coast which lies west of the peninsula of Florida, the Ohio states have ready intercourse, by the Mississippi river; but with the region of the east of that peninsula, they are destitute of all adequate means of commercial and social connection. Here then is a great desideratum, which can be supplied in no other manner than they by the contemplated Railroad.

Starting, perhaps from more than one point on the Ohio river, in the state of Kentucky, this [rail]road should stretch nearly south; and branching, when it enters the Carolinas and Georgia, to reach their tide-waters at several different places. Taking Cincinnati as a city intermediate between Maysville and Louisville, and Charleston as intermediate between Wilmington, in North Carolina, and Augusta, Georgia, the [rail]road might be said, more especially, to connect Cincinnati and Charleston, and may for convenience in this report, takes its length and designation from those two cities....

The distance between Cincinnati and Charleston, on a straight line, is about 500 miles, which would probably require a road of 700 miles. South Carolina, however, has already made a rail-way, 135 miles in length, to Hamburgh, on the Savannah river, opposite Augusta, nearly in the direction of Cincinnati; and the contemplated rail-road to Paris, in Bourbon county, Kentucky, exactly in the course of Charleston would have a length of about 90 miles, thus, leaving but 475 miles to complete this new and most important communication, between the interior and the sea-board of the south....

It may be said, however, that the central part of the Cincinnati and Charleston [rail]road would run through a country thinly inhabited, and furnishing little aid, either in the construction of the [rail]road or in swelling the amount of transportation upon it. But why is it so sparsely populated? Manifestly, in part, because of all portions of our common country, it is the most inaccessible and the most destitute of facilities for the exportation of its iron, salt, coal, tar, turpentine, and other natural productions. To wait, therefore, for a denser population, as a condition for commencing a great work of internal improvement, which only can augment that density, would be to wait for the development of an effect before resorting to the only cause than can produce it. Let the [rail]road be executed and an instantaneous impulse will be given to improvement to the region. If, however, it were too sterile for such a result to occur, no argument against the project could arise from that fact, for the undertaking is necessary to the reciprocal exchange of the production of the states penetrated by its extremities, in which respect it would be similar to the Philadelphia and Pittsburgh route, which, in a part of its course, passes over uninhabited mountains, and still facilitates an immense trade between east and west....

No public work could contribute more powerfully to our national defense. Establishing a direct and rapid communication, between northern and southern frontiers of the United States, separated, unlike the eastern and western, from the dominions of foreign nations by narrow sheets of water only, it would afford facilities for the transportation of troops, munitions of war, and military sustenance, from the center to the borders, or even from one frontier to the other, with unexampled rapidity; thus, favoring a concentration, requisite to national defense in time of war, which could not otherwise be effected; and which would present a new triumph of civilization over barbarism, by making civil public works, an efficient substitute for standing armies and powerful navies, which exhaust the resources and endanger the liberties of a nation.

But the most interesting and affecting consequences that would flow from the execution of this enterprise, would be the social and political.

What is now the amount of personal intercourse between millions of American fellow-citizens of North Carolina, South Carolina, and Georgia, on the one hand, Kentucky, Ohio, Indiana, and Illinois, on the other? Do they not live and die in ignorance of each other; and perhaps, with wrong opinions and prejudices which the intercourse of a few years would annihilate forever? Should this work be executed, the personal communication between north and south would instantly become unprecedented in the United States. Louisville and Augusta would be brought into social intercourse; Cincinnati and Charleston neighbors; and parties of the pleasure start from the banks of Savannah for those of the Ohio river. The people of the two great valleys would, in summer, meet in the intervening mountain region of North Carolina and Tennessee, one of the most delightful climates in the United States; exchange their opinions, compare their sentiments, and blend their feelings—north and south would, in fact, shake hands with each other, yield up their social and political hostility, pledge themselves to common national interests, and part as friends and brethren.

Finally, the immense summer throng of visitors which annually go up to the north, along the sea-board, would be made still greater, and turning westwardly, through the states of Virginia, Maryland, Pennsylvania, and New York, spread over the northern center of the United States, to the shores of the lakes and upper Mississippi; concentrating on their return in the valley of the Ohio; having seen what they now never see, and made acquaintance with what at present is unknown to them, the very heart of the Republic. On the other hand, the people of the north would, in autumn and winter, pour down upon the temperate plains of the south, in turn, studying their political, civil, and literary institutions, participating in their warm hospitality, catching a glow of southern feeling, gratifying their curiosity, and return enlarged in their patriotism and enriched in their knowledge of our common country: Thus this traveling, along, would, at no distant day, reimburse the expenditure by which it was created, while it would unite with the ties of business, in confining with a new girdle, states which are now but loosely connected, and thereby contribute powerfully to the perpetuity and happiness of the Union.

Railroad from the Banks of the Ohio River to the Tide Waters of the Carolinas and Georgia. Cincinnati: Printed by James & Gazlay, 1835.

Reader Reflection

1. *To facilitate community connections what infrastructure barriers need to be addressed or overcome? How would you do that?*
2. *What is needed to promote tourism in your community? What is the benefit to the local economy to learn about others from distant communities/countries?*
3. *In what ways, if at all, does your community seek out connections with distant communities? Identify one possible connection and list the potential benefits.*

2.28 Why Communities Should Value Medical Schools

I shall proceed to display more fully the interest which the community has in the prosperity of medical institutions. To enumerate the various advantages conferred upon society by well-regulated medical schools may be considered superfluous; as they fall upon us unceasingly, from the moment of our birth to that of our dissolution. Like the genial effects of heat and light, we cease, however, to observe them, because they are uninterrupted. Having become imperceptibly blended with the other elements of our happiness, we are unconscious of their influence, and without the aid of analysis, they continue through our whole lives, like secret benefactors, to administer to our comfort unobserved and unappreciated. There are occasions on which this analysis should be made; and in pleading the cause of an infant seminary, I should be recreant to its interests, did I not call upon the enlightened community, on whom it must rely for the aliment of its growth, to inquire how far their happiness is connected with the medical profession.

Most of the occupations in society reflect upon it merely the limited advantages of their immediate application to its necessities. The profession for which I have the honor to plead is capable of dispensing a wider range of benefits and blessings. Its proper object is the cure of diseases, but in becoming qualified for this, its members are prepared to render many other important services. Imbibing in the course of their collegiate studies a taste for the cultivation of letters and science, and being afterwards received into the bosom of every society, they contribute powerfully to infuse the same taste, where it might otherwise be wanting. Impelled by necessity, as well as inclination, to continue the prosecution of sciences which benefit mankind through other channels than the profession of medicine, they not infrequently become the authors of discoveries and inventions which in their application to the common purposes of life, materially augment the sum of its enjoyments;—or, devoting themselves to the cultivation of one of the auxiliary sciences, increase the number of its facts; enlarge its boundaries; and elucidate its principles, or apply them with new success to useful and ornamental purposes. This is especially the case in a new country, where literature and philosophy are not yet self-existent; but must rely for protection and cultivation upon an alliance with the learned professions. It is in such a country that the usefulness of a scientific physician spreads widest through society, and his character displays, comparatively, its broadest and brightest disk. But the chief purpose of the life and labors of the physician, as already intimated, is the prevention and cure of disease; and this object is of the greatest magnitude, whether we consider it in reference to the preparation which it imposes on him; or to the countless multitude of blessings which it confers on society.

An Inaugural Discourse on Medical Education. [Delivered at the Opening of the Medical College of Ohio in Cincinnati, November 11, 1820.] Cincinnati: Looker, Palmer, and Reynolds, 1820. 23, 24, 25.

READER REFLECTION

1. *Drake is making the case for support for a new medical school and hospital in this address. Fundamentally he is asking the following questions: "What is the benefit of institutions on society? Are the benefits continuing?"*

2. *Should this assessment of institutions be a practice done in each community? For example, what is the benefit of this institution? Is it still needed? Is it achieving its original aim? Does its aim need to change? Is the institution being socially accountable?*

3. *Consider: Are there any core institutions in your community that are taken for granted? What are the hidden benefits of a medical school and hospital that need to have a light shone on them?*

✱ 2.29 ORGANIZE MEDICAL SCHOOLS TO BE UNDER THE SOVEREIGN POWER OF THE STATE AND LOCALLY MANAGED

No one can dispute the propriety of placing Medical schools under the supervision of the law; and rendering them amenable to the sovereign power of the state. It will avail but little, however, that they are thus authorized, if that power does not govern them with liberality, vigilance, and wisdom. They should be regarded, not as private, but public incorporations; designed for the benefit of society, rather than of the individuals who compose the faculties. A medical professorship is indeed a public office; and should be filled or made vacant from no other motive, than the general good. No claims for admission, but those founded on talents and general fitness, should ever be allowed; and the discovery of a failure in these, and this only, should be regarded as a justifiable ground of dismissal. The principle of rotation in office should never operate to effect the removal of a competent professor.

When a State is about to institute a medical college, and subsequently, it should have special regard to several points:

1. The Location. The proper site for such a school is a populous city. Uncommon talents in the professors may secure, for a time, the prosperity of a school in any situation; but misplaced, it is liable, like a plant in a barren soil, to perish or decay, when committed to unskillful or indolent keeping.

2. The Endowment. Some kind of revenue, or an actual appropriation of adequate amount, should always accompany the charter; not as a bonus to professors, but to afford them the means of research and illustration [teaching].

3. A Hospital. This should be as ample as possible, and so planned and regulated, as to be made a clinical school, and a school of morbid anatomy. The rights and duties of professors and pupils should be clearly specified; and both made so comprehensive, as to secure for the sick, the best possible attendance; while they, in turn, should repay society and the profession, for the charity they receive, by the benefits which their cases can be made to confer on the pupils.

4. The Supplies for the Anatomical Hall. Exhumation should be prohibited, under the severest penalties, [and] rigorously enforced; but all who are found dead in the streets or fields, who die in hospitals, poor houses, houses of correction, jails, and penitentiaries, and not claimed by friends, and taken away to be interred at their own expense, should be delivered to the professors of the college. This would abolish the practice of disinterment [grave-robbing], which, otherwise, must and will continue, until other sources of supply are opened. The opposing demands and denunciations of society, on this subject, indicate that the present is, indeed, but the age of transition from a lower to a higher grade of civilization. Society, in former times, did not require anatomical knowledge, in whom it entrusted the limbs and lives of its members; at a future period, it will afford to its medical guardians the means of acquiring the knowledge it demands.

5. The Trustees. These should be chosen for their qualifications. They should not only be men of talents, intelligence, and literature; but, from taste, inclined to devote themselves to a faithful execution of their stewardship. Above all, they should be men of honor and impartiality—tolerating in their hearts neither prejudice nor prepossession—and conducting the institution with a sole view to the public good. A part of them should be physicians, but not of the city in which the college is established, lest collisions in professional business, between them and the professors, should disturb the harmony of the institution.

6. The accountability of the trustees is to those from whom they derive their authority. This should be made as rigorous as possible. The trust being strictly eleemosynary [dependent on charity], should be confided to no board of trustees any longer than they are found to render it beneficial to those for whom it was granted. Annual detailed reports should be required form the Board, accompanied by reports from the Faculty, and these should be submitted to the scrutiny of select and competent committees, with instructions to investigate closely, and report impartially, on the state of the institution; all which should finally be published, together with the new acts of fostering or corrective legislation, which they may have suggested. By these means, abuses would be detected, and a powerful motive infused into the trustees, to act with the skill, moderation, and justice, which befit those who should be accountable to public opinion, as well as the laws.

Thus founded and governed Medical Schools, are a blessing to mankind, and reflect the highest honor on the governments from which they emanate.

"Legislative Enactments." In *Practical Essays on Medical Education and the Medical Profession in the United States.* Cincinnati: Roff & Young, 1832. 89–91.

READER REFLECTION

1. *Institutions that serve the public good endure. Trustees are stewards to keep the public good as the primary mission of such institutions. What advice does Drake give here for the trustees of public institutions? Should this advice be changed, and, if so, how?*

✠ 2.30 THE BEST CLINICIANS IN THE COMMUNITY SHOULD TEACH IN MEDICAL SCHOOLS

Medical colleges, on their present plan, were not known till since the revival of letters, in Europe. For two or three centuries, they were few in number, and chiefly sustained by the genius and labors of individual professors; of whom [Herman] Boerhaave, [Albrecht van] Haller, and the first [Alexander] Munro, maybe cited as illustrious examples. The 18th century augmented their number, and established their importance; but it was reserved for the 19th to multiply them to an unprecedented degree, and show that they may be composed, in part, of men who the pride of science would, formerly, have pronounced unfit for such a lofty and difficult duty.

In the United States, the number [of medical schools] at the close of the last century did not exceed three: it is now at least 15, and others are annually springing up. This extraordinary increase may be ascribed, in part, to the great number of State sovereignties which make up our confederacy, each of which, instead of the federal government, grants college and university charters; and is ambitious to rival its neighbors in the number, if not the excellence of its institutions. But another cause is equally operative. This is want of due care in the selection of professors; by which the standard of professorial excellence is depressed to a level that brings the office within the reach of unqualified aspirants; and offers to mediocrity of talents, a degree of encouragement which no age or nation ever before held out.

Did the best talent of the American profession find its way into our numerous schools, it cannot be doubted that they would be able be sustained; but truth and justice require me to say, that this is not always the case; that every part of the union presents men of loftier genius, sounder learning, and purer eloquence, than many of those, whom the trustees of our different institutions, from time to time, select as professors.

"Medical Colleges." In *Practical Essays on Medical Education and the Medical Profession in the United States.* Cincinnati: Roff & Young, 1832. 45–46.

READER REFLECTION

1. *In your field what is the process for selecting the most talented individuals to be involved in teaching and training the next generation?*
2. *Are the best, most talented in your community involved in teaching and training?*
3. *What are the barriers to attracting talented teachers to your community?*

⊠ 2.31 WORK WITH THE LEGISLATURE TO CREATE AND SUPPORT A MEDICAL COLLEGE

Whereas, society at large is deeply interested in promotion of medical and surgical knowledge; and whereas, the students of medicine in the State of Ohio are so distant from any well regulated college as to labor under serious disadvantages in the prosecution of their studies; therefore,

SECTION 1. Be it enacted by the General Assembly of the State of Ohio, that there be established, in Cincinnati, a college for instruction in physic, surgery, and the auxiliary sciences, under the style and title, "THE MEDICAL COLLEGE OF OHIO."

SECTION 2. Be it further enacted, that Samuel Brown, Coleman Rogers, Elijah Slack, and Daniel Drake, with their associates and successors, shall constitute the faculty of professors of said college, and, as such, are hereby created and declared the body corporate and politic, in perpetual succession, with full power to acquire, hold, and convey property for the endowment of said college, contract and be contracted with, sue and be sued, plea and be impleaded, answer and be answered unto, defend and be defended in all courts and places, and in all matters whatsoever; provided, that no part of the estate, either real or personal, which said incorporation may at any time hold, shall be employed for any other purposes than those for which it is constituted. And, provided, also, that the revenues arising from the property, which the said incorporation shall be entitled to hold shall never exceed the sum of five thousand dollars per annum.

SECTION 3. Be it further enacted, that the faculty of said college may devise and keep a common seal, which may be altered and renewed at pleasure.

SECTION 4. Be it further enacted, that the officers of said college shall be a president, vice-president, registrar, and treasurer, who shall be elected by the professors out of their own body, once in two years, at such times, in such manner, as they appoint; which offers shall hold their places until their successors are chosen.

SECTION 5. Be it further enacted, that two-thirds of the members of the faculty of said college shall constitute a quorum for every kind of business, and, when thus assembled, shall have full power and authority to make, ordain, and resolve all by-laws, rules, and resolutions, which they may deem necessary for the good government and well being of said college; and the same when deemed expedient, to alter, change, revoke, or annul, establish such additional offices and appoint such officers and servants as they may think requisite for the interest of said college; also to create alter or abolish all such professorships or lecturers, when thus dismissed, shall cease to be members of the corporation; provided, that no professorship shall be created or abolished, nor any professor lecturer be elected or dismissed, without the concurrence of three-fourths of the faculty.

SECTION 6. Be it further enacted, that the faculty of such college shall have power and are herby authorized to confer the degree of medicine, and grant diplomas for the same under the seal of the corporation.

SECTION 7. Be it further enacted, that, until the faculty of said college shall direct it otherwise, there shall be established the following professorships: first, a professorship of the institutes and practice of medicine; second, professorship of anatomy, third, a professorship of surgery; fourth, a professorship of material medica; fifth, a professorship of obstetrics and the diseases of women and children; sixth, a professorship of chemistry and pharmacy.

SECTION 8. Be it further enacted, that, until the faculty of said college shall make different arrangements, the following person shall be and are hereby appointed professors, viz.: Daniel Drake, Professor of the Institutes and Practice of Medicine; Samuel Brown, Professor of Anatomy; Coleman Rogers, Professor of Surgery; Elijah Slack, Professor of Chemistry and Pharmacy; and, until the said faculty shall hold an election for officers, the following are hereby appointed, to-wit: Daniel Drake, President; Coleman Rogers, Vice-President, and Elijah Slack, Register and Treasurer.

SECTION 9. And be it further enacted, that this law shall be subject to such alterations and amendments as any future legislature may think proper.

Ohio Laws: Acts of the General Assembly. Vol. 17. Chillicothe: George Nashee, 1819. 37–40. [Substantially drafted by Donald Drake. Passed on January 19, 1819.]

READER REFLECTION

1. *In a democratic society every generation works with, influences, and assists the governing bodies to advance initiatives to improve the public good. What motivates individuals to get engaged in this way? How does an individual get engaged in the process?*

2. *Consider the long-term consequences on the community and the lives of individuals of creating such learning institutions through the state legislature.*

✠ 2.32 Create a Teaching Hospital

"It is in hospitals, the lectures on practical or clinical medicine must be delivered. To hear those and witness the cases to which they relate, would be an object every student who might attend the Medical College. The fees of admission for these purposes would go into the treasury of the hospital; and, as the professional attendance on the sick would, under this regulation, cost but little, the revenues thus accruing would, after a few years, become adequate to all the expenses of disease among this unfortunate and degraded class of our population. We should then make them do in sickness, what they did not perform in health—support themselves. The price of their exhibition, moreover, would be paid by persons from a distance, whose other debasements during a residence here, would become a source of positive benefit to the city.

The Legislature of Louisiana, in the true spirit of benevolence, has proposed the different Mississippi states the erection of hospitals for the sick boatmen on the various waters of that great river. On this subject, the Governor of Ohio has received a communication from the Governor of Louisiana, which will be transmitted to the next legislature. I cannot for a moment doubt, that this honorable body will make an appropriation for an object involved so deeply the prosperity and reputation of our state; and Cincinnati, as its commercial metropolis, would, of course, be the spot where the establishment would be erected. It will not be necessary, however, that the state should maintain a distinct and independent hospital for this object. Their efforts might, with great propriety and advantage, be united with those of the guardians of our poor and the Faculty of our College—the state supplying the means of erecting a common edifice, the city maintaining the police and expenses, and the college supplying it gratuitously with medical assistance.

A poorhouse with shops and gardens might be made part of the same establishment, and the whole confided to the care of a single board of managers. It is sufficiently apparent, however, that such a work cannot be accomplished without a general union of means; a hearty cooperation of efforts; a liberal and considerate course of legislative policy; and, above all, a deep and general conviction of its necessity and benefits. If this happy communion of feeling and design could be effected, our city would soon be graced with a house of charity, in which the unfortunate, when diseased, would find refuge and relief; and the people of the whole state an asylum for the insane, that would wipe away the disgrace of confining them in the cells of our common jails; while our students of medicine, enjoying more ample opportunities of improvement would become benefactors, instead of the scourges of society."

By this extract we see the origin of our hospital [1820]. In the second month of the first session of the school, a bill was drawn up by one of the Faculty [Drake], and laid before the trustees of the township of Cincinnati. It proposed a union of the college, the township, and the state, in the establishment of a public charity. The trustees wisely gave it their sanction, and united with the Faculty in a memorial to the General Assembly, which had already been informed, by Governor [Ethan Allen] Brown, of the application from the Governor of Louisiana. When I carried the memorials and bill to the legislature, they met with opposition; but, after a month of laborious explanation and personal effort, the bill became a law. The state, having in view the relief of her sick boatman, gave a small sum of money to assist in the erection of a house, and pledged, forever, half the auction duties of the city, toward the support of the patients. The township was to supply the remainder, and the professors of the college were to be its medical and surgical attendants, with the privilege of introducing their pupils for clinical instruction— the fees of admission constitute a fund for the purchase of chemical apparatus, anatomical preparations, and books for the college. Such was the second step [creation of the charter of the Cincinnati Hospital and Lunatic Asylum] taken by the State of Ohio for the promotion of medical education, the chartering of the college being the first.

An Introductory Lecture, at the Opening of the Thirtieth Session of the Medical College of Ohio. Cincinnati: Morgan and Overend, Printers, 1849. 13–14.

READER REFLECTION

1. *In 1820, joining public service institutions with teaching and training was innovative. It is a model still in use today. Consider examples other than teaching hospitals in your community. What public service institutions are/could be coupled with teaching and training?*
2. *What makes such collaborations work? What did Drake do as summarized in this selection to accomplish the creation of a "teaching hospital"?*

2.33 RECOGNIZE THE NECESSITY OF HOSPITALS

The necessity for Hospitals in the Valleys of the Mississippi and the Lakes, for the relief of those engaged in our commerce, and also, of travellers, had been perceived from the infancy of the Western settlements; but it was left for a benevolent physician, of the State of Missouri, Dr. Cornelius Campbell of St. Louis, to set foot the project of urging the General Government to establish them. The Committee have given to this subject the serious attention which its importance demands, and have come, unanimously, to the conclusion, that it should be earnestly and respectfully pressed on the attention of Congress....

From the absence of such hospitals, at short intervals, many valuable lives have been lost, that might have been preserved, if timely aid had been administered. This is sometimes done, by the skill and humanity of the steamboat commanders; but the flat boats are, generally, unprovided with requisite medicines, and on board of both, it is not uncommon for persons to sicken and die, without medical assistance; the boat still keeping on her way, and only stopping to deposit the remains of the deceased, in some new village, or underneath the trees of the forest.

Your committee are not prepared to speak definitely of the number and locality of the hospitals, which an extension of the trade of the West will ultimately require; nor even to point out with precision the points, where, at this time, they are most needed; but they venture to indicate the following, as the places where they are now wanted; New Orleans, Natchez, Memphis, St. Louis, Louisville, Cincinnati, Pittsburgh, Buffalo, Cleveland, and Detroit.... With such, or even a less number, no sick person on board a steamboat or schooner would suffer longer than one or two days before he could be lodged in a hospital where the early applicant of medicine might preserve his life, and permit him to prosecute his voyage, without being able to command the requisite medical advice, whereby many valuable lives would be saved, and the prosperity of our commerce greatly promoted.

The location, erection, and support of these hospitals are not likely to be accomplished by the different States; for justice requires, that the advantages they would afford should be reciprocally enjoyed, and, therefore, that they should not only be erected at the same time, but in such places as would combine the whole into one great system of national charity; neither of which could be accomplished without such negotiations between the States interested, as are not contemplated in the Federal Constitution.

"Report on the Necessity for Hospitals in the Valleys of the Mississippi and the Lakes for the Medical Convention of Ohio." *Western Journal of Medical and Physical Sciences* 8 (1834): 461–462.

READER REFLECTION

1. *Some initiatives to improve the public good are national in their coordination and execution. Drake saw this and advocated for the development of a system of strategically placed hospitals for seaman/boatman who were transient and suffered for lack of care as they were involved in supporting interstate commerce. What are the emerging needs to the public good that require our attention and potentially national coordination? Who is engaged in those needs today with whom you could get involved?*

2.34 LEVERAGE THE VOICE OF A LARGER ORGANIZATION TO ACCOMPLISH NEEDED CHANGE

1. Resolved, That, in the opinion of this [Medical] Convention [of Ohio], the sessions of the different Medical Schools throughout the Union are too short and they ought to be extended one month, and the students required to stay to the end of the term.

2. Resolved, That, the number of Professorships is too few, and that ampler provision should be made for teaching Physiology, Pathological Anatomy, Phar-

macy, and the Natural History of Medicines, Botany, Comparative Anatomy, Meteorology, Medical Jurisprudence, and Mental Physiology.

3. Resolved, That, if practical, our Medical Schools should be so organized as that Students in their first course would have their attention chiefly directed upon special Anatomy, Physiology, Chemistry, Pharmacy, and the other elementary branches; and their second upon Pathological Anatomy, Therapeutics, the practice of Physic, Surgery, and Obstetrics.

4. Resolved, That in admitting Candidates to examination for degrees, a stricter regard than is at present shown should be had to their preliminary education.

5. Resolved, That, the practice of graduating young men before they are 21 years of age should be abandoned.

6. Resolved, That, no Pupil ought to be graduated before the end of four years from the time he commenced the study of Medicine.

7. Resolved, That, if the various Schools of the Union were to send representatives to a meeting at some central point, to confer together, many of their existing defects, by a simultaneous cooperative effort might be successfully remedied and that we respectfully recommend such a Convention to be held. Till then it would not be practicable nor should be expected that any single institution will attempt the reforms which are here proposed.

8. Resolved, That, the corresponding Secretary be instructed to send a printed copy of he proceedings of this Convention to all the Medical Institutions of the United States, with a letter calling the attention of their Professors to these Resolutions.

Committee on Defects in the Organization and Administration of Medical Schools. *Journal of the Proceedings of the Medical Convention of Ohio, at Its Second Session, Columbus, Ohio, January 1, 1838.* Cincinnati, 1838. 17.

READER REFLECTION

1. *A single individual writing an opinion piece can have impact, but a collected body of experts working together and publishing a similar set of comprehensive recommendations can have even greater impact due to the "brand" of the organization. What society or organization has a respected voice that you could work with to accomplish needed reform or change in your discipline or field? What kind of reforms do you think need to be addressed?*

✖ 2.35 Emerging Careers: Enhance the Training and Responsibility of the Apothecary

The profession of the Apothecary should receive attention from our legislatures. The practice of keeping and putting up their own medicines is going rapidly out of fashion among the physicians of all the cities and larger towns of the Union. In consequence of this, the compounding of prescriptions is passing from students of medicine, to the clerks and shopkeepers of druggists, most of whom, as well as their operatives, are mere merchants, almost entirely ignorant of the branches of science connected with the business which they follow; and equally destitute of classical learning.

They who put up physician's prescriptions should be acquainted with Botany, Materia Medica, Chemistry, and Pharmacy, and possess such a knowledge of the Latin language, as would enable them to decipher, with correctness, what is sent to them. If ignorant in these respects, they are, perpetually, liable to make mistakes, which may defeat the objects of the physician, and even destroy the life of the patient.

The law should, indeed, not only require apothecaries, who undertake to compound the recipes of the profession, to be qualified, for that nice and important duty; but, also, to file and preserve the manuscripts sent to them, that a proper responsibility may be established, and the blame of errors, by which the sick may be seriously injured, fixed on those who commit them. Without this skill and precaution, the lives of patients are in perpetual jeopardy.

"Legislative Enactments." In *Practical Essays on Medical Education and the Medical Profession in the United States.* Cincinnati: Roff & Young, 1832. 93–94.

Reader Reflection

1. *With the advance of knowledge and technology, new careers are created. What new careers are emerging, and what special training programs, requirements should be created to equip the individuals in those careers?*

✖ 2.36 Meet a Community Need: Formation of the Cincinnati Eye Infirmary

Dr. Drake, one of the editors of this journal, in a recent visit to the east, has made the necessary arrangements, and is about to establish in this city, an infirmary for diseases of the eye—both clinical and surgical. They will be modeled after the excellent institutions of a similar kind recently established in New York, by Dr. Delafield and Rogers, and in Philadelphia, by Dr. Hays....

According to the practice pursued in the eastern infirmaries, those who are unable to pay, will be operated on gratuitously.

"Eye Infirmary." *Western Medical and Physical Journal* 1 (1827): 126–127.

By the aid of a number of benevolent citizens of Cincinnati, Dr. Drake will be able to defray the expense of poor persons from the country, while they are under treatment in the city. To such his professional services will be offered gratuitously. His regular prescribing days are Wednesdays and Saturdays, between the hours of 10 and 1 o'clock; but in urgent cases he may be consulted at anytime.

"Cincinnati Eye Infirmary." *National Republican and Ohio Political Register* 5 (November 16, 1827).

READER REFLECTION

1. *When trying to create a solution for your community consider Drake's approach: Identify a need, explore how others are addressing the problem in other communities, engage local citizens in the effort to support, create the plan to execute, and then monitor the results.*

✠ 2.37 ADVOCATE FOR A SCHOOL TO INSTRUCT THE BLIND

It must gratify every friend of humanity, and raise a feeling of laudable pride in the heart of every citizen of Ohio to hear of the successful operation of the school for the Education of the Deaf and Dumb, at Columbus. The effects already produced in the short space of five years would do credit to an older community than ours; and are an encouraging earnest of the many blessings it will confer on those who are born to perpetual silence, in the midst of a noisy world.

Among the various advantages that result from such a humane institution, is this: that it awakens the tenderness of the people at large, and predisposes them to new enterprises of beneficence. Under this conviction, we think it a favorable time, to present to the consideration of our General Assembly, of the Profession and Society at large, the establishment in Columbus, of a sister Institution for the Education of the Blind.

The number of these unfortunate persons, we mean to include those only who are children, or were such when they became blind, is far greater than is generally supposed. For several years, we have professionally, been devoted, in an especial manner, to the treatment of Diseases of the Eye, and every month has presented us with new evidences, of the great number of blind children and youth, within our own State. Many of these were born blind, and might, of course, be cured; but a much larger number became so, in infancy or childhood, from inflammation of the eyes, and their cases are generally irremediable. A large portion of these are children of poor parents, and belong to the country, where sore eyes prevail more than in the towns, and are too often subjected to no medical treatment, till incurable blindness is produced. Thenceforth, the child becomes a permanent charge on its parents or friends—often on the township—and passes its life, not only deprived of the enjoyments of sight, and all the benefits of intellectual education, but with the painful consciousness, of being a perpetual burden on those about it; while, if educated, its happiness would be greatly increased, its moral faculties and affections ameliorated, and its bodily powers made available, to its own support.

The education of the Blind, like that of the Deaf, cannot be conducted at home, even when parents, from their wealth, have the necessary leisure. Specific methods and qualified teachers are indispensable; and if such could be obtained, in sufficient numbers, and all who have blind children had the means of compensation, the progress of the pupil would be in no degree equal to what it is, when associated in a school, with others, laboring under the same infirmity.

It is then, obviously the duty of every State, to institute and support a school for the education of the Blind; in which not only their intellectual and moral faculties should be cultivated, but they should be taught some mechanical occupation, of a useful kind, and the prosecution of which would enable them to earn a livelihood, and raise them from a state of dependence on their friends or the community. Such institutions have existed for some time, in Europe, and have lately been established in Pennsylvania, New York, and Massachusetts, with the most beneficial results. As yet, there is not one in the Valley of the Mississippi, where the proportion of poor blind children, is greater, perhaps, than in any other part of the Union. Ohio has nearly one third of the population of the Great Valley, and why should she not be the first to institute this noble charity? Having nearly completed, and brought into productive operation, several magnificent public works, her present resources are every way adequate to the humble, but still dearer object, of instructing those unfortunate children, who, without such advantages, can never participate in the enjoyment which every citizen derives from contemplating these honorable achievements.

"School for the Instruction of the Blind." *Western Journal of Medical and Physical Sciences* 7 (1833): 483–485.

READER REFLECTION

1. *Are there subgroups in your community who have limitations, disabilities, or obstacles that prevent them from reaching their full potential? What is being done on their behalf? Is more needed? Is the local or state government involved? Are there best practices in other communities that could be adapted and implemented?*
2. *What is the impact on community cohesion when a community cares for its own?*

2.38 COMPETITION AS A DRIVER OF IMPROVEMENT

One third of the population of the United States is in the Valleys of the Mississippi and the Lakes, while the whole region has but two schools, one of which has been pronounced by the profession of the state whose name it bears, and by a large majority of the physicians of the city, in which it has been in operation for fifteen years, and by its own TRUSTEES, to be utterly defective—a sentence which is confirmed by the small number of its pupils. Is there no need, then, of reform, or of a better school? Shall there be fourteen medical schools among eight millions of people in the other states, and a ban put upon those who would have more than two for four millions in the West, when one of these two is so unattractive as to be the night or tenth school in the Union, in the number of pupils? Kentucky, with but two-thirds of the population of Ohio, gave to her own school, last winter, one hundred and twenty students, at least double the number of all the paying pupils in the Ohio School from every quarter! I state as fact, that a medical gentleman declared, at the Columbus convention of physicians in January, that he knew, in the county in which he resided, and in an adjoining county, no less than eight students of medicine, who were in attendance on lectures in eastern schools! And this too after our state has given thirty-six or thirty-seven thousand dollars for the establishment of a college at home. Shall it be said that this college has not yet attained to puberty? It may not in functions, but certainly has in years. Early and rapid development is the constant effect of the warm moral and social climate of the West; and where there is any thing to come forth we see it unfolded betimes. Thus, the third class of Kentucky comprised 138 pupils, which is more than the Ohio School has yet numbered. The sixth class of the former reached 282—the twelfth of the latter 200 less! When the 282 assembled, they found themselves in what has been the bar room of a tavern!—there was no public edifice, the state had not, has not since, given but $5000; while all the circulars of our college have set forth the magnificence of Ohio, and the magnitude and splendor of the college edifice, the attractive front of which, has more than once been engraved, at the expense of the state, and sent abroad in books, and newspapers, as a substitute for the fame of the professors. Unfortunately for those who relied on this artifice, students attend medical schools to be instructed, not to sit in splendid edifices; to listen to the eloquence of professors—not to admire the beauty of columns, which adorn the empty and echoing halls. The Jefferson Medical College was instituted in 1825, five years after the Medical College of Ohio; without any endowment from the state of Pennsylvania; and under the very walls of the venerable and popular university, which is honored with the name of the state, and cherished by the wealth and moral power of the city; and still, with all these disadvantages, it has already attained to three times the number [of students] of the Ohio College, placed in a spot more favorable to the building up of a great school, than almost any other in the Union.

"Reform of the Medical College of Ohio." *Western Journal of Medical and Physical Sciences* 9 (1835): 169–203.

READER REFLECTION

1. *A monopoly can create advantages that lead to self-interest, exploitation, and even loss of service or quality. Competition from a rival organization or business can actually raise the level of quality or service and also lower cost—increasing value. Why is it that competition often leads to adversarial relationships rather than realizing a competing organization actually is the stimulus to make the other better?*

2. *Facts are stubborn things. How can you use facts to call out self-interest, exploitation, and the like, in a public institution?*

▩ 2.39 Indifference and Division among Members of a Community Hinder the Establishment of Institutions

A majority of the people of Cincinnati are emigrants from every civilized country, and did not come hither to cultivate literature, as commerce—to erect scientific, as manufacturing establishments. Their emigration, moreover, was neither in colonies, nor in concert; hence they arrived strangers to each other, in a strange land, without a more specific common object, than the pursuit of fortune and happiness. In such a population, although the individuals, like those of Cincinnati may be highly estimable, there can be but little devotion to literary and scientific projects; and still less of that active and harmonious effort, by which alone they can be reared and sustained. It is not surprising, therefore, that the obvious importance of a medical school to a city should have been generally overlooked; and that till lately very few of our citizens should have manifested a more active interest in its success, than to give it a passing benediction.

From this prevailing indifference has sprung its most overwhelming troubles; for while the people of Lexington gave munificently to a rival institution, those of Cincinnati contributed nothing to this; and while public indignation at that place would have fallen upon the most distinguished man in society if he had traduced either the school or the humblest of its professors, public unconcern, in this city, has tolerated the sneers of the most insignificant; and encouraged an opposition which in a well organized society would have been promptly and indignantly subdued. This opposition, which began to show itself soon after the school was projected, originated with a part of our practitioners of medicine, and had for its object the destruction of the whole scheme. Their motives could not be mistaken. A successful medical school would increase the number of scientific competitors in the city; and also raise the standard of excellence in the profession, to a degree which their natural dullness and confirmed indolence in study, would find unattainable. The project must therefore be destroyed; but to declare war against it, might incense the community—it was as yet a mere project, and would sink if the projector should be overthrown. Thus originated the hostilities in which I have been so deplorably involved for the last three years. I might have ended them at any time, by abandoning the enterprise; and thus established an enviable reputation for humility and contemptibleness; instead of being denounced as ambitious, militant, and outrageously persevering; but from an unaccountable obstinacy I selected the latter.

In the course of this protracted combat, my character was assailed, both openly and covertly, with every missile which these gentlemen had the ingenuity to invent or the desperation to wield. The vain-glorious and indiscreet ventured into the newspapers; the more cautious and timid thought it safer to animate the flighty combatants, and infuse poison into the minds of the community by private conversations. Between the two orders of assailants the magazines of billingsgate were emptied; and the quivers of calumny exhausted of all their arrows. In the community this war of words excited the indignation of the few; but the many found nothing in it save diversion; and when a repetition of the same sounds began to pall upon their ears, they expressed themselves "tired of the doctors' quarrels," and hoped they would soon be at an end. It was the smaller number only, who took the trouble to ascertain that from the first I had acted on the defensive; who perceived the aim and effect of these continued aggressions; who had the experience to foresee that it might prevent the establishment of a medical school in Cincinnati—the public spirit to deplore that so useful a project should be wantonly destroyed—or the justice to defend its projector from the fire of the enemy, while laboring to fix its foundations. This, however, was at length accomplished.

A Narrative of the Rise and Fall of the Medical College of Ohio. Cincinnati: Looker & Reynolds, Printers, 1822. 17–19.

Reader Reflection

1. *In creating institutions expect indifference and even opposition. What allows an individual to endure and work through these challenges?*
2. *Have you ever faced such opposition? What allowed you to get through it and see an initiative succeed?*

2.40 Philanthropy Makes a Difference

A disease so wide-spreading and mortal as Epidemic Cholera, must of course have a powerful remote cause, but what it is, has not yet been discovered. The ingenuity of the profession has suggested several, but strong objections lie against the whole....

If such a cause does not exist, why is the world now trembling at the geographical progress of an Epidemic, as uniform in its symptoms as small pox, and as fatal in its termination as the plague? The existence of such a cause must, I think, be admitted. Whether it will ever be discovered is extremely doubtful. Meanwhile, philanthropy and science should exert themselves in correcting or removing all the conditions that cooperate with it in the work of human destruction, and thus disarm, if they cannot slay the monster.

A Practical Treatise on the History, Prevention, and Treatment of Epidemic Cholera, Designed Both for the Profession and the People. Cincinnati: Cory and Fairbank, 1832. 25, 50.

READER REFLECTION

1. *Cholera was poorly understood and there was no formal research support in place. The microscope had just been in use opening up a whole new area of research in the microscopic world. Drake proposed that all the data on causation pointed to the "animalcular hypothesis"—an organism likely so small, that living in fluids, it can only be seen by the microscope. It would be twenty-two years later that the agent causing cholera was discovered, but the information not more widely translated to prevent cholera for thirty more years.*

2. *How has philanthropy been and continues to be critical to the advancement of science? What happens when philanthropy is limited or minimal?*

2.41 INSTITUTIONS NEED ASPIRATIONAL GOALS TO GUIDE IMPROVEMENT

My missions are: to salute you as pupils of the College; and on behalf of its Trustees and Professors, to welcome you within its walls, and give you the assurance, that whatever may be practicable will be done for your instruction and comfort.

Of the prospective and probable value of our labors to these ends, it is not my intention to speak; but I may remark, that whether it be much or little, a willing and earnest cooperation on your part, will be indispensable to your improvement. It will therefore, be expected of you to be punctual in your attendance in the College and Hospital, orderly in your deportment, courteous to each other, respectful to your teachers, temperate in your habits, and unwearied in your devotion to study....

I must declare to you that I stand ready to pledge the remainder of my active life, and all the humble talents with which the Creator has endowed me, to her [the College of Medicine] future elevation; and where I to put up the prayer of Hezekiah, for length of days, it would be to devote them to her aggrandizement; and, for the pleasure of seeing her halls overflowing with inquiring pupils, attentively listening to ardent, learned, and eloquent professors. With this pledge, those who watch over her welfare, and those who govern the Hospital which she caused to be erected, are now silently mingling theirs; while you, I trust, are resolving that your own lives shall spread abroad her fame. Thus will she rise, and gracefully move onward and upward, until she stands in beauty and honorable rank, among her distinguished sisters of the Union—the pride of her sons, and a blessing to society.

An Introductory Lecture at the Opening of the Thirtieth Session of the Medical College of Ohio, November 5th, 1849. Cincinnati: Morgan and Overend, Printers, 1849. 3, 16.

READER REFLECTION

1. *As institutions and organizations are launched, leaders often have a vision and aspirations to guide them to success. In those institutions and organizations where you are involved, do they have a vision and aspirational goals to guide them? Can you articulate them?*

Writer

"An Able and Philosophic Writer"

"An old man's pen, once turned up on the days of his youth, is a siphon, with one end in the great reservoir of the past, and the other on his paper, through which the current will flow until the vessel is exhausted."

—Daniel Drake, *Pioneer Life in Kentucky: A Series of Reminiscential Letters from Daniel Drake, M.D., of Cincinnati to His Children*

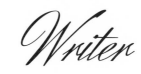

3.1   *Count the Cost to Allow Your Powers to Unfold and Blossom*

3.2   *Exercises to Become a Better Writer*

3.3   *The Difficulties of Finding Time to Write*

3.4   *A Writer Creates an Outlet for the Words*

3.5   *Take an Interest in Learning to See and Describe What Surrounds You*

3.6   *Descriptive Writing: The First Settlement of Cincinnati*

3.7   *Descriptive Writing: A Child's Rich Experience on a Nature Walk*

3.8   *Descriptive Writing: The Beauty of the Great Lakes*

3.9   *An Author Struggles to Arrange and Sequence the Presentation of Information*

3.10 *First Medical Publication:* Notices Concerning Cincinnati *(1810)*

3.11 *Starting a Journal: Editorial Policies of the* Western Journal of the Medical and Physical Sciences

3.12 *Suggested Rules for Preparation of Medical Papers*

3.13 *Editorial: "Medical Hoax"*

3.14 *Editorial: "Clerical Encouragement of Quackery"*

3.15 *Editorial: "Progress of Science"*

3.16 *Traveling Editorials: Sharing the Plan and Inviting Others to Contribute Information*

3.17 *Vision and Plan for a Practical Medical Reference:* Principal Diseases of the Interior Valley of North America

3.18 *Introducing Medical Topography*

3.19 *Proposing a Needed Textbook in Pathology*

3.20 *Advocacy: The Pursuit and Acquisition of Knowledge Pays Rich Dividends and Is Worthy of Support*

3.21 *Advocacy: Public Letters in Support of Henry Clay for President (1824)*

3.22 *Advocacy: Calling Out the Need for Educational Reform*

3.23 *Advocacy: The Need for Reform of Medical Education*

3.24 *Defense after Dismissal from the Medical College of Ohio*

3.25 *Use of Humor: A Novel Site for Smallpox Vaccination*

3.26 *Writing to Combat Quackery: "The People's Doctors"*

3.27 *Poetry: "My Mother"*

3.28 *Poetry: "Hymn for My Mother's Funeral, November 10th 1831"*

3.29 *Private Journal: Reflecting on Marital Love after My Wife's Death*

3.30 *Poetry: "The Lover's Winter Visit"*

3.31 *Poetry: "Hymn"*

3.32 *Poetry: "Funeral Hymn for the Sixth Anniversary of His Wife's Death"*

3.33 *Letters: Remembering Those We Have Lost*

3.34 *Letters: The Reality of Death*

Chapter Three

— *Drake was a prolific writer who published seven books and boasted a bibliography of over 700 citations.*

— *He became the first medical author west of the Alleghenies with the publication of* Notices Concerning Cincinnati *in 1810. He was also the editor of one of the earliest medical journals for twenty-two years.*

— *While Drake is best known as a medical researcher and essayist, he was also a poet, letter-writer, and memoirist that pursued writing as a personal passion. Not all of his works were published.*

✠ AUTHOR INTRODUCTION

In Drake's time the written and spoken word were the primary methods of communication, and thus, words mattered. Being a good speaker and writer was the primary means for shaping public discourse and building a reputation. These literary and oratory skills were necessary for learning and growing and for improving and achieving. For Drake good writing meant writing with "simplicity, conciseness, clarity, and purity [accuracy]." To do so required practice.

Learning to write was a primary goal for Drake, and he adopted specific methods to teach himself how to write well. First, he read widely with a notebook on hand to record specific passages and his reactions to them. Early on a dictionary was often by his side to help him grow his extensive vocabulary. In taking notes he sought to translate the works of others into his own words. Second, he taught himself to accurately observe nature and describe what he saw. Third, he also practiced writing by rewriting the sections from the works of great authors, a suggestion he took from Benjamin Franklin's autobiography.

Fourth, he created written summaries of the works he was reading. Fifth, he taught himself to translate works from foreign authors. Sixth, he wrote essays and gave public addresses on various topics. He was attentive to how words sounded when spoken, and many of his addresses include frequent punctuation to facilitate the pauses used for an oral presentation. Seventh, he became an editor of a medical journal that required him to critique the works of others and also allowed others to critique his work. With all these exercises and habits, he created time for writing in the midst of frequent interruptions from the demands of medical practice, teaching, and his personal life. He often wrote late into the night, and for his longer books, he used the school breaks to create longer blocks of uninterrupted time. His approach is a model for anyone who desires to improve writing skills.

Over his career he used different types of writing for specific purposes and occasions. As a naturalist he was most comfortable with descriptive writing. His first book, *Notices Concerning Cincinnati*, and his second book, *Statistical Notes on Cincinnati*, were intended to describe the rich resources of the region and in turn stimulate interest in others to settle in the "emerging western country." As an editor of the *Western Journal of the Medical and Physical Sciences* he contributed scientific articles, editorials, announcements, obituaries, and selections from his travel journals. Series of thematic articles in the journal were eventually assembled into books (for example, essays on medical education or studies of cholera). He wrote newspaper articles to advocate for specific political causes, social reforms, and to defend himself when attacked by jealous competitors. He could use humor, satire, and sharp polemic to drive home his message. As a popular speaker he wrote addresses on specific topics of the day (temperance, discipline, the arts, the value of institutions, philanthropy) or special occasions (for example, the anniversary of the founding of Cincinnati). He opened the medical school year with introductory addresses during his thirty years as a teacher. His major medical work, the two-volume *Systematic Treatise, Historical, Etiological, and Practical, on the Principal Diseases of the Interior Valley of North America*, took over a decade to write and presented his conceptual framework for describing the diseases and how they varied by topography and as a result of specific factors (ethnicity, diet, climate). He was a historian who wrote memoirs about the early beginnings of Cincinnati and its medical profession. For his family he wrote letters, poetry, and a commemorative journal (unfortunately his son destroyed the full-length manuscript of the journal, saving only brief selections).

The selections in this section offer a sample of some of the above, but the other selections in this book's other sections also illustrate Drake's style of writing and the extent of his use of the written word to make an impact on the world around him and contribute to his enduring legacy.

✠ 3.1 COUNT THE COST TO ALLOW YOUR POWERS TO UNFOLD AND BLOSSOM

What high capacious powers lie folded up in man;

How far beyond the praise of mortals may the eternal growth of nature to perfection half divine expand the blooming soul?

What pity then should sloth's unkindly fogs depress to earth her tender blossom; choke the streams of life, and blast her spring!

Medical Diary; or, Common Place Book. HMD Collection, 2931123R. National Library of Medicine, Bethesda, MD. January 22, 1806.

READER REFLECTION

An early example of Drake's writing, this was the opening page of his diary of his first set of studies in Philadelphia in 1806 under the great physicians of the day: Drs. Benjamin Rush, Caspar Wistar, Philip Physick, Benjamin Barton, and William Shippen. At age twenty he had already recognized the human potential that is unleashed by industriousness.

1. For you to bloom in your career what are the threats that could choke "your streams of life"?

2. This is an example of keeping a "commonplace book," a personal notebook recording events, notes, observations, and reflections. Get in the habit of keeping such a journal.

✠ 3.2 EXERCISES TO BECOME A BETTER WRITER

The young physician should write as well as read. *He should study with his commonplace book by his side,* especially when engaging works which he does not expect to peruse a second time—and make them such references, or, from them such extracts, or, of them such abridgments, as may same advantageous. It is a most useful exercise to abridge and rewrite such parts of the great authors, as relate to some interesting subject, and place them in juxtaposition, for the purpose of comparison or contrast. He should sometimes epitomize entire works, for the mere value of the exercise in professional composition; and to the same end translate, largely, from all the languages he may cultivate. *He ought carefully to record his own observations and experiments*; not in diffuse and inaccurate style, but with precision and perspicuity.

The epoch of professional life now under consideration is the *time to perfect those habits of observation*, which begin in our pupilage. Every clinical case ought to be a study and nothing connected with it should be overlooked. I never knew a skillful practitioner who was not an astute observer. Whatever may be a physician's judgment, he should not be confided in, if obtuse in his powers of observation. To arrive at correct results, the first and greatest requisite is to have *correct data*; which can only be acquired by accurate and patient observation.

He should from time to time write essays and dissertations on speculative topics and at a subsequent period subject them to a rigid criticism. By these various exercises, he will, at length, *acquire a habit of expressing himself with facility and clearness*, if he should never attain to elegance; while these repeated attempts at arranging and connecting facts, *will have strengthened his reasoning powers, and given him habits of method*. It is lamentable to see how few of us write well, that is, with simplicity, conciseness, and purity. The fault lies quite as much in the neglect of practice and composition, as in the want of previous education. Neither will do alone; but of the two, the former is, perhaps, the more injurious.

"Studies, Duties, and Interests of Young Physicians." In *Practical Essays on Medical Education and the Medical Profession in the United States.* Cincinnati: Roff & Young, 1832. 63–65.

READER REFLECTION

1. *Drake suggests a set of specific exercises (at least seven) to improve your writing. What are they? Do you use any of them?*
2. *According to Drake, to become a skilled writer it is essential that you become a skilled observer. Do you agree or not?*

3.3 THE DIFFICULTIES OF FINDING TIME TO WRITE

I have not written to you, and some others, for a longer time than I ever kept silent before. The reason for this Mr. M. will understand more fully, perhaps, than any other of my correspondents, as his experimental knowledge of the perplexities of authorship could not have left him ignorant on that point. But even Mr. M. is not fully prepared to imagine, in what a degree of embarrassment I have been immersed for six months past, unless he was obliged to study the elements of the sciences to which they belong, to make a dozen applications for a fact, which might be answered in as many words, to exchange the inkstand and pen for the Lancet and gallipot [small pot made of earthenware or metal used by pharmacists] every hour in the day, and above all to confront boldly a succession of pertinacious duns. About all this, and more, he could not experimentally know to what I have been subjected this summer. In the midst of such difficulties and distractions, greater proportion, I suspect, then those in which Dr. [Samuel] Johnson composed his folio dictionary, nothing but absolute necessity could have kept me to the course.

Excerpted from letter [circa 1815] cited in *The Life of Daniel Drake,* by Edward Mansfield. Cincinnati: Applegate & Co., 1855. 110.

Reader Reflection

This letter was written after Drake was finishing his book Natural and Statistical View; or, Picture of Cincinnati and the Miami Country. *The book uses multiple primary sources to confirm facts and achieve accuracy. But it caused Drake, in the midst of a busy career fraught with interruptions of medical practice, great difficulty to write, as alluded to in this letter.*

1. *With every project there are hidden costs. Consider some of your projects and identify some of those hidden costs.*

3.4 A Writer Creates an Outlet for the Words

At the close of my letter to your sister Echo two days ago, I declared that I should and would dismiss from my mind the matters, a part of which were embodied in its fifteen pages; but when I ordered them out, they would not go. Even while before my class, engaged in delivering an extemporaneous lecture on pleurisy, they still hovered round; and as soon as I left the university, began to gambol before me as friskily as a troop of fairies in the nectary of the blue violet. I then saw that I had no resource but to drown them in ink, and lay them out on paper to dry, like butterflies in the cabinet of the entomologist. This I have now undertaken to do; but as drowned fairies are not so far as the living, nor dead butterflies so beautiful as those which are swarming in the beams of the summer sun, so, I am quite sure, you find my delineations very far inferior to the images which memory has recalled into existence. And still there are relations in life—those of parents and children, of husband and wife, of brother and sister, of friend and friend—which give importance and even sanctity, to the smallest events and humblest actions; and hence I feel that you, and the others for whom these words are intended, may find an interest in them sufficient to justify the expenditure of time which their presentation may require at my hand.

Pioneer Life in Kentucky: A Series of Reminiscential Letters from Daniel Drake, M.D., of Cincinnati to His Children. Edited by Charles D. Drake. Cincinnati: Robert Clark & Co., 1870. 19–20.

READER REFLECTION

1. *Where does the nagging impetus to express your thoughts in written form originate? An accompanying desire is to make such thoughts interesting, worthwhile, and memorable. Discuss why these desires are common among writers.*
2. *Discuss a time when you just had to write something down.*

✖ 3.5 TAKE AN INTEREST IN LEARNING TO SEE AND DESCRIBE WHAT SURROUNDS YOU

It is not, however, among these important classes [of birds], that the greatest number of novelties in the zoology of this region can be found. The obscure and imperfect animals that swim in our lakes and rivers, infest our morasses, dimple our pools, and swarm among the flowers of our fields; those which, like our white perch, are remarkable only for their nutritious qualities; or, like the great rattlesnake of our museum, for living whole months in captivity without the aid of any nutritious substance; or, like the minute insects, which sometimes overcloud our atmosphere, and exhibit an unwelcome example of the distribution of a small portion of life among a multitude of beings, apparently to augment the sum of its power; those animals, in short, which delight the historian, rather than the poet of nature, have been least studied by us, and at the same time are not only most numerous, but contain the greatest portion of what are peculiar to this country. The more noble and perfect animals traverse extensive continents, and become citizens of the world, while the imperfect are frequently limited to a narrow range, and seldom extend their migrations beyond a single district. An abundant feast is, therefore, in reserve for those who delight to study animated nature in every form, and can equally admire her attributes, whether humble or exalted.

An Anniversary Discourse, On the State and Prospects of the Western Museum Society. Cincinnati: Looker, Palmer, and Reynolds, 1820.

READER REFLECTION

1. *As a writer the world around you is an abundant feast. The ability for observing and describing the world are valuable assets in any career. How does one learn to observe and describe? How would you rate your ability to observe and describe?*
2. *Describe a time when, through careful observation, you noticed something important that no one else had noticed before.*

3.6 DESCRIPTIVE WRITING: THE FIRST SETTLEMENT OF CINCINNATI

When Major Doughty came from Fort Harmar it was uncertain which of the three points in the Miami settlement ought to be selected as a permanent military post—we have not now, the time to inquire into all the reasons which led to the choice of Losantiville, but its greater exemption from river inundation than either of the other settlements should have been sufficient. The government directed that a fort should be built in this place, and the spot selected was on the upper plain near its margin east of Broadway. Third Street produced passes through The Esplanade. The Fort was erected in the summer and autumn of 1789. It was of hewn logs and had a quadrangular figure with four bastions the southwestern on the spot now occupied by the bazaar, and the great massive gate opening to the south. The stockade of pickets extended north in the direction of fourth Street. A well was dug in the graveled esplanade from the center of which, a tall flag staff supported the waving stripes and stars—an object on which the exposed families of the pioneers delighted to gaze. In the course of the autumn several hundred additional troops arrived as an expedition against the Indians was in contemplation. Between the fort and the river, on a part of the 15 acres reserved by the general government when [John] Symmes received his patent, a great number of sheds were erected for the combination of the artificers [craftsmen] and commissaries. On 29 December 1789, a year and three days after the first landing, General [Josiah] Harmar, previously having made Fort Harmer at the mouth of the Muskingum his headquarters, arrived at Losantiville with 300 additional soldiers. He immediately took possession of the Fort and named it Fort Washington, in honor of the father of his country.

"Memoir of the Miami Country 1779–1794" [an unfinished manuscript for the Western Historical Society]. *Quarterly Publication of the Historical and Philosophical Society of Ohio* 18 (1923): 2–3.

Reader Reflection

It was important to Drake to share with his community its history.

1. *How well do you know the history of your community? Is there an opportunity for you to be involved in recording local history?*
2. *How does studying local history add value to your community?*

3.7 Descriptive Writing: A Child's Rich Experience on a Nature Walk

When the sensible and benevolent parents or teacher combines a visit among the various objects of the natural world, as the reward he would bestow for obedience, or great effort at labor or study, he presents the highest sensual gratification, which God has place at his disposal....

What joy instantly beams from every [child's] countenance! and how strikingly must each contrast his happy lot with that of the offender who is left behind in confinement! How directly must he associate the reward with the observance of duty which procured it! What bustle of preparation ensues, what contempt of bad weather, and bad roads, what feelings of young enterprise and impatience to be gone, start up in every palpitating heart! Spring is unfolding her beauties—the air is genial—the light now and then interrupted by a passing cloud, raised high in the heavens, and threatening no shower to damp their ardor—the meadow lark, perched on the crag of a decaying stump, and the cat-bird in the thicket, raise their notes, and the urchins hasten to the spot and put the songsters to flight—the squirrel is then treed, and lies flat and quiet on the limb, while club after club passes harmless by; one boy, more aspiring then the rest, attempts to climb the trunk, becomes dizzy, and slides sheepishly down over its rough bark, ashamed to catch the eye of her, whose admiration he sought to win, and half provoked at the shouts of merriment which his failure called forth, to die away the next moment, when some straggler announces a new violet, raising its timid head through the faded leaves of the preceding autumn! Then the steep hill, and the race of boys and girls to its top, the descent to the new and shaded hollow beyond, the jumping of the little brook, with the young gallantries it brings forth; lying down to drink, by some thirsty boy, and another, filled with mischief, pushing his face into the water from behind; the discovery of a petrifaction and the gathering together, to wonder at its form, and struggle for its possession! Now, the admiration of the half expanded buds, and a transient comparison of those of different bushes! Then, the union of all the boys, under some leader, designated as it were by instinct, to roll over the rotten log, and the discovery of a harmless little snake; the instinctive impulse to kill, the haste and uproar of the execution, and the terror of the girls, who, afterwards, see a snake in every stick they are about to tread upon! The continuance of the ramble, till it reaches the dogwood, the red-bud, and the buckeye, with their blooming limbs, the climbing, the breaking, the throwing down, and the scrambling below, till all are loaded to their heart's content, and by some new route they return home, fatigued and hungry, to tell of the great discoveries, and boast of great deeds. And where has been the parent or teacher throughout this scene of pleasure? If at the post of duty, in the midst of every pastime, and attentive to every opportunity of doing good; explaining each object, pointing out every relation, disclosing the properties and qualities of each attractive plant, separating the different parts of its flower, and teaching their names and connections, lecturing on the woods, commenting on the thunderbolt which destroyed the ash, but passed instinctive and harmless over the beech tree, by its side; calling attention to the backwardness of vegetation on the north side of the hill compared with the south, and teaching that it is the effect of differences in heat; thus inspiring a love of knowledge in the young mind, when excited by pleasures of the body, disclosing to it some of the most beautiful laws of nature, and directing the young heart up to her great and benevolent Author.

Such are the fruits of an excursion made in such manner as to gratify the senses of childhood, and none can fail to see in them, a reward that may be pressed into the service of school and family government with the happiest immediate results, and the most admirable effects upon the future character of the objects of our affection.

"Discipline: Discourse on the Philosophy of Family, School, and College Discipline." *Transactions of the Fourth Annual Meeting of the Western Literary Institute and College of Professional Teachers.* [Meeting held in Cincinnati October 1834.] Cincinnati: Josiah Drake Publisher, 1835. 43–44.

1. Descriptive writing is a good place to start as a writer. Use all your senses to capture informa-
tion to translate into a description of a meal, a walk in nature as Drake does here, or a new
experience. Introduce a life lesson into the description to create a second layer of meaning.

2. Note the exclamatory style used here. What style of writing best fits your manner of description?

✠ 3.8 DESCRIPTIVE WRITING: THE BEAUTY OF THE GREAT LAKES

When the observer directs his eye upon the waters more than the land, and the day is fair with moderate wind, he finds the surface as variable in its tints, as if clothed in a robe of changeable silk. Green and blue are the governing hues, but they flow into each other with such facility and frequency, that while still contemplating a particular spot, it seems, as if by magic, transformed into another.

But these midday beauties vanish before those of the setting sun, when the boundless horizon of lake and land seems girt around with a fiery girdle of clouds; and the brilliant drapery of the skies paints itself upon the face of the waters. Brief as they are beautiful, these evening glories, like spirits of the air, quickly pass away; and the gray mantle of night warns the beholder to depart for the village, while he may yet make his way along a narrow and rocky path, beset with tufts of prickly juniper.

Having refreshed himself for an hour, he may stroll out upon the beach, and listen to the serenade of the waters. Wave after wave will break at his feet, over the white pebbles, and return as limpid as it came. Up the straits he will see the evening star dancing on the ruffled surface, and the lagging schooner flapping its loose sails in the fitful land breeze; while the Milky Way–Deaths Path of the Red Man, will dimly appear in the waters before him....

Surrounded by such scenes, the traveler begins to realize that he is a stranger, when suddenly a new phenomenon appears and fixes the conviction. Every object becomes more visible, and, raising his eyes, he beholds the heavens illuminated with an Aurora Borealis, where he reads in fantastic characters of light, that he is, indeed, a sojourner in a strange land, and has wandered far from his friends and home in the sunny regions of the south.

The Northern Lakes: A Summer Residence for Invalids of the South. Louisville, KY: J. Maxwell Jr., 1842. 28–29.

1. *Imagine you are a tourist guide and you wish to make a place attractive for others to visit and experience. Try your hand at writing about that place. What would you want visitors to experience?*

✂ 3.9 AN AUTHOR STRUGGLES TO ARRANGE AND SEQUENCE THE PRESENTATION OF INFORMATION

A book of this kind [*Natural and Statistical View*] should contain whatever it is desirable to know, concerning the spot of which it professes to treat. The relations of a town with the surrounding country, are an essential part of its history, and cannot be understood without studying both. The author is by no means so confident that he has adopted the best mode of exhibiting this information; and then giving it a formal distribution under the heads which have been employed for geographical delineations of greater extent, he does not expect to escape the charge of a precise and finical devotion to method; but with the hope, that the opportunity it afforded of disposing the materials in that state of arrangement which will facilitate a reference to any particular subject, he felt no disposition to pursue a different plan, merrily to avoid so harmless a criticism. A more ample field for animadversion will perhaps be found in the examination of his style. 'Tis true, the merit of a topographical work, composed chiefly of facts and observations, does not depend all together on the choice and collocation of the words in which it is expressed; but still it is a sacred duty of every writer to improve, rather than corrupt his language. The author performs, therefore, merely an act of justice to himself, when he declares that the imperfections in his style have arisen either from indolence, nor contempt of public opinion, but from causes which lie beyond the sphere of his control; and at the same time, it is equally due to the reputation of his fellow townsman, that he should protest against the reception of this performance as a fair specimen of their literature.

Natural and Statistical View; or, Picture of Cincinnati and the Miami Country. Cincinnati: Looker and Wallace, 1815. vii–viii.

READER REFLECTION

Drake's intent was to describe the multiple positive relations of the surrounding country with

Cincinnati in ways to promote the development of the region. He was concerned how he might be critiqued, so he sought to diffuse some of the anticipated criticism.

1. *Consider the effort required if every writer felt it was his duty to improve, rather than corrupt, the language.*

✠ 3.10 First Medical Publication:
Notices Concerning Cincinnati (1810)

And now, having successfully presented myself, as the first pupil and the first graduate of the town [Cincinnati], I may add, as completing the medical history of its first 21 years, that I was also its first medical author; having in 1809 written for distribution a pamphlet on its Etiology and Diseases under the title of "Notices Concerning Cincinnati." It was printed in the office of the Reverend John W. Browne, and set by a worthy man at this moment, perhaps, among you, Mr. Sackett Reynolds, then an apprentice in the office. I cannot say of it as professor Woodhouse said of his introductory lecture after delivering it the twelfth time that I find new beauties in it every year; yet we must not entirely overlook the "day of small things." For this is the only specimen of our medical literature, for the first half of our city and professional existence.

"Early Physicians, Scenery, and Society of Cincinnati." *Discourses Delivered by Appointment before the Cincinnati Medical Library Association.* Cincinnati: Moore and Anderson, 1852. 57.

Reader Reflection

1. *What are the first or great published works about your community? What impact did they have during their time?*
2. *What was your first publication? If not yet, what thoughts do you have about writing for publication?*

✠ 3.11 Starting a Journal: Editorial Policies of the
Western Journal of the Medical and Physical Sciences

It is not without regret, that he [the Editor] finds himself thus situated; as his editorial duties were, of themselves, sufficient to occupy most of the time, which professional engagement left at his disposal. Inured, however, to hard labor, and deeply interested, as he has become, in the success of the undertaking, he is far from cherishing a feeling of discouragement. The following contributions are requested:

1. Rare or singular cases of disease. To report all cases would be impractical and absurd. To report the successful only, is uncandid. Cases which go to the suggestion of a new principle or rule of practice; which either weaken or sustain a disputed point; which terminating unfavorably, may serve as a warning to the profession; and finally, those which occur with exceeding rarity may always be published with advantage to others, and credit to the reporter.
2. New forms of disease, depending on causes, either discovered or unknown.
3. Annual epidemics.
4. Brief or synoptic reports, consisting of a sort of account current with the weather and diseases, of the different seasons.
5. Accounts of new medicines.
6. Experimental treatises on our native medicinal plants.
7. Chemical and therapeutic accounts of our mineral springs.
8. Comparative histories of the diseases of the Negroes and whites.
9. Facts for an estimate of the peculiarities, which the diseases prevailing on board of steamboats of the Western and Southern waters may present.
10. Reports on the diseases in our penitentiaries.
11. Detached facts, in clinical medicine, which may be proper for insertion under the head of original, miscellaneous intelligence.
12. Notices of the discovery in the west and south, of such minerals, as are in anyway employed in pharmacy.

The Editor would not, however, absolutely restrict his correspondence to new facts; in as much as he believes that on many subjects a new arrangement of old ones, is imperiously required; he would be happy, therefore, to receive and publish essays and dissertations and on subjects in the profession, provided they develop either new principles or new practical maxims.

"To the Physicians of the Western States." *Western Journal of Medicine and Physical Science* 2 (1828): i–vi.

Reader Reflection

1. *One of the ways to have an impact on a community is through serving as an editor and regularly publishing articles by others. Drake was thoughtful about what information would be important to capture that would identify key principles or be of practical use to the reader, to the profession, and to the community. How do you decide on what important principles or information of practical use to include in your communications?*

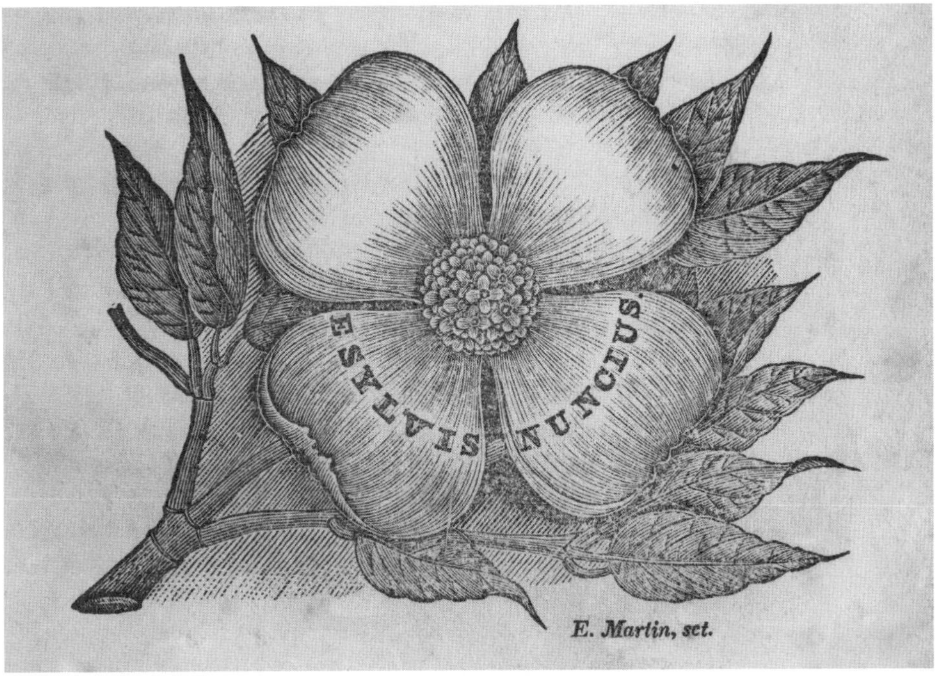

The dogwood flower, the symbol of Drake's journal, *Western Journal of the Medical and Physical Sciences. Digital copy courtesy of the Henry R. Winkler Center for the History of Health Professions.*

3.12 Suggested Rules for Preparation of Medical Papers

The first excellence is *truth*. Everything that is published in a journal of medical science, should as far as possible, be divested of error; for it may all, sooner or later, influence the treatment of the sick, whose lives might be jeopardized, in consequence of perversions or suppressions of the truth. The next great requisite is *perspicuity* [clarity]: that what the writer has observed and thought, may be readily and clearly comprehended. The next is *conciseness*: which many readers would in reality place at the head of the column of good qualities: and it cannot be denied, that they would have much reason on their side; for the quantity that is published, in the journals, and detached works, of the present age, is really enough to deter the timid and indolent from all reading. *Originality*, is another important property, which should be never wanting. Mere learning, and laborious rumination of that which has been masticated by others, will neither advance the interests of the profession, nor satisfy readers' good sense. Finally, those who write for medical journals should not consider the minor *rules of composition* beneath their attention. If advanced in years and reputation, their example will be authoritative, and should, therefore, be a good one: If young, they should seize every occasion to improve themselves in the art of writing. Indeed, no member of the profession, either high or low, should consider himself at liberty to disregard the *laws of orthography* [spelling], *etymology, syntax, and collocation* [word position] in anything which he presumes address to his brethren. Lastly, in mercy to editors and compositors, he should write or procure to be written in an unaffected and *legible* hand, without which, he has, in fact, no guaranty that the printed will be a correct copy of his written communication.

"To the Physicians of the Western States." *Western Journal of Medicine and Physical Science* 2 (1828): i–vi.

READER REFLECTION

1. *As a writer do you seek to improve? What are you doing to get better at your writing?*
2. *How would you assess your writing using Drake's outline: truthful, free of error, clear, concise, original, stylistically and grammatically correct?*

3.13 EDITORIAL: "MEDICAL HOAX"

During the early part of last month, two or three of our younger physicians made a few Galvanic experiments on a criminal recently hung in this city, by which some slight muscular contraction was excited, though not quite as usual in such cases.

On this state of fact a correspondent of one of our newspapers proceeded to construct a report which, as we have been told, for we did not read it, represented this criminal as raised to his feet and made to walk about the room, performing a variety of pantomimic gestures. We perceive by the newspapers, that this report has been regarded as authentic, and as it stated that another might be looked for in our Journal, we feel it a duty to make that which we have just penned.

We cannot but regret, that our newspaper press should so often give utterance to fabrications intended to deceive the public. What is a hoax but a falsehood? And what is there in the publication of a falsehood that can be approved? If our brethren of the political press cannot make their papers interesting to their readers, without imposing on them the creations of imagination as facts relating to passing events, they would do well to abandon the profession for some calling in which the price of bread is not the sacrifice of veracity, or the practice of imposture.

"Medical Hoax." *Western Journal of Medicine and Surgery* 3 (1841): 399.

READER REFLECTION

1. *The press should have a high standard for veracity. What happens to a press that does not have a high standard for veracity and spreads falsehood? What is the impact on the community?*
2. *What is our responsibility to prevent or respond to falsehood or hoaxes?*

✠ 3.14 EDITORIAL: "CLERICAL ENCOURAGEMENT OF QUACKERY"

We can scarcely open a newspaper, without meeting with the advertisement of one or more quack medicines, recommended and avouched by clergymen. Now such is the confidence of the mass of the people in their spiritual pastors, that these certificates have in them a power, even greater than the forged testimonials of eminent, deceased physicians, so often seen appended to the same advertisements. Such being the case, we would respectfully ask our clerical friends, to whom we attribute no bad motive in this manner, whether they ever reflected on the mischief they do to the community, by these recommendations? Do they not know, that if a nostrum be *inert*, a reliance upon it may destroy life—if *active*, that while it may relieve or even cure a few, it will kill many more? We would charitably believe, that most of these certificates are given without due reflection. The majority of them are for cough mixtures, balsams, boluses, or lozenges, which are presented as infallible remedies, without reference to the nature of the disease in the lungs, by which the cough is produced. But the diseases of the lungs are of a various kinds—requiring different modes of treatment—and what may cure one patient may kill another. If a clergyman, then, has seen a quack medicine relieve an individual, he is not justified in generalizing, and commending it to all who may, from coincidence of a single symptom, fancy themselves in the same condition.

Medicine is an inductive science, the basis of which is a knowledge of the structure and functions of the human body. He who builds on this foundation, rests his superstructure on a rock—all others build on sand. How many clergy-men understand anatomy and physiology beyond Dr. [William] Paley's *Natural Theology*? We suspect very few. We ask these respected brethren, what they mean by orthodoxy? Is it not a full acquaintance with the letter and spirit of the Bible, and a faithful adherence to both? Now medicine, so to speak, has its orthodoxy, which consists in a profound knowledge of the principles of science, and a reliance on them to guide us in practice, as the divine relies on the doctrines of the Bible to guide and govern him in preaching. If some ignorant layman, but super-ficially acquainted with that divine revelation and unimbued with its spirit, were to advertise a new exposition of its doctrines—a sort of patent mode of securing Heaven—what would our clerical friends say, if physicians who had never made the Bible a study, were to certify to the truth and efficacy of such a pretended discovery? They would undoubtedly warn the people to beware. It would be a dereliction of duty for them to remain silent; and we, on the other hand, feel, that duty in reference to the health and temporal welfare of the community, commands us to speak out, in words of warning to the people and of rebuke to such spiritual leaders, as travel out of their profession, to enlist under the banner of quackery in another.

"Editorial: Clerical Encouragement of Quackery." *Western Journal of Medicine and Surgery* 4 (1841): 235–236.

READER REFLECTION

1. *Why does every generation have some who are gullible and undiscriminating and fail to recognize when they are being led astray? Why do some people disregard truth and follow the alluring voice of the quack?*
2. *How do you combat the quack? Who is responsible for this?*

3.15 EDITORIAL: "PROGRESS OF SCIENCE"

It must gratify the friends of sound and solid science to learn, the *College of Professional Teachers*, at their late meeting in our sister city of Cincinnati, requested "doctor" Rosenstein, the famous homeopathist, to enlighten them and the good people of that city, with a lecture. Such a thirst for knowledge is highly auspicious. We presume the "doctor" administered to each member of the College, the true homeopathic dose, of a hundred thousandth part of a grain of truth, mingled in a glass of gall and wormwood against the *regular* profession. But why should the College have limited itself to the homeopathists, when...others were at hand, and ready to expound their respective systems? Such partiality we cannot approve; it is at war with the true democracy of science, and, if persisted in, will undoubtedly bring the College into disfavor with the friends of those improved systems, which are more numerous than the advocates of homeopathy. In this way the College will render itself unpopular and diminish its influence. Perhaps, however, it has appointed committees to make reports at the next meeting, on those reformed methods; and thus obviated the charge of partiality. If so, very well; but lest it should have regarded any of the other new improvements as worthy of encouragement, we take the liberty of presenting the first rude draft of a preamble and resolutions, to be adopted at the next annual meeting of the College.

Whereas, in the opinion of this College, established to promote sound learning and exact science, the world has been held in bondage for three thousand years, by a succession of men calling themselves the disciples of Hippocrates, who profess to have made discoveries concerning the laws of the human body and the means of preventing and curing its diseases, whereby they have imposed on the unwary, to the great detriment of their constitutions; and whereas a number of original geniuses in modern times, have made important hygienic discoveries, which are rejected by the aforesaid disciples of Hippocrates, through jealousy and envy of said discoveries, and from malice prepense towards society; and whereas it is the duty of this College to foster neglected genius, not less than to humble the pride of science, therefore

Resolved, That a committee of seven members, not physicians, be appointed to make a report, to the next session of the College, in favor of the following newly discovered systems of medicine for the people to wit:

1.   On Hanemannism, or Homeopathic doctoring;
2.   On Mesmerism, or Magnetic doctoring;
3.   On Cornstalkism, or Indian doctoring;
4.   On Radicalism, or Root doctoring;
5.   On Brandrethism, or Pill doctoring;
6.   On Thompsonianism, or Steam doctoring;
7.   On Guineaism, or Negro doctoring.

Resolved, That said committee be instructed, to warn the community against the pretended discoveries of Hippocrates, Celsus, [Giovanni Battista] Morgagni, [William] Harvey, [Thomas] Sydenham, [Marie François Xavier] Bichat, [Benjamin] Rush, and others of like kind, and against the schools of medicine in the United States, where their writings are received as authority.

Resolved, That the members of this College will, henceforth, patronize some one of the aforesaid seven wise men; preferring, however, the last, from the well known curative powers of a seventh son.

Resolved, That should any other *College of Professional Teachers* attempt to forestall this, in the proposed reform of the medical profession, it shall be the duty of the "Executive Committee" to appoint a special meeting of the College, that it may, by early action, not lose the honor of achieving what it is the first to undertake.

Resolved, That in all future meetings of the College, the practisers of the aforesaid seven new systems, shall be entitled to seats; and that such of them as cannot write their names, shall be allowed to subscribe the constitution by making their marks.

"Editorial: Progress of Science." *Western Journal of Medicine and Surgery* 4 (1841): 400–402.

READER REFLECTION

1. *How effective is the use of satire in shaming individuals, corporations, or organizations to correct an error or improve? Try using satire to effect change.*

⬙ 3.16 TRAVELING EDITORIALS: SHARING THE PLAN AND INVITING OTHERS TO CONTRIBUTE INFORMATION

Traveling Editorials. This phrase admits of no less than three applications. It may mean editorials for the benefit of travellers; editorials of such excellence and interest, that they will travel far and wide among the profession; or editorials written while traveling. It is in the last sense that we use the expression....

Last summer, when, in visiting the shores of the [Great] Lakes, we commenced the series of medical travels which have now been resumed. In their prosecution, it is our object: 1st to acquire a knowledge of the modifications of our climate, from the Lakes to the Gulf, with their influence on the constitution of the people.

2nd To note the various geological and topographical conditions, which may be supposed, directly or indirectly, to occasion or prevent diseases. 3rd To observe the diet, drinks, occupations, and manners and customs of the inhabitants, as predisposing to, producing, or preventing diseases prevalent in their respective localities, as can be drawn from them by personal interviews. 4th To collect facts for a comparative estimate of the physiology and pathology of the Europo-American, the Indian, and the Negro.

Our field of observation extends from Michigan to Florida, and from the western slopes of the Alleghany mountains, to Missouri, Arkansas, and Iowa.

Such is the enterprise on which we have entered at an advanced period of life [age fifty-eight], though some of the activity and feeling which belong to earlier years. Should we not live, or otherwise fail, to achieve it, we have the satisfaction to believe that our researches may still be of some benefit to the profession, inasmuch as we can scarcely fail to record many valuable facts, which might otherwise be lost, and which by some abler hands may be presented to the public.

In addressing these paragraphs to our readers, and all other medical gentlemen within the extended region we have designated, we are actuated by an earnest desire to secure their co-operation. Without it, a failure is inevitable. With it, some degree of success may be regarded as almost certain. Therefore, we respectfully solicit their co-operation.... We take this method to request such of our readers as reside in those States, to prepare for us, in writing, such transcripts of their experience as may be fit materials for our projected work. We would extend this request to all who practice medicine in the various States west of the Alleghenies, in the hope, that they will perceive the necessity of their co-operation, and that they will forward to us, at no distant time, the facts which are requisite to a full history of our most important diseases.

"Traveling Editorials." *Western Journal of the Medical and Physical Sciences* 7 (1843): 239–240.

READER REFLECTION

1. *Writing a letter appealing for assistance is a common necessity. What makes a good and effective appeal letter that leads to results? What does Drake do here?*

✠ 3.17 VISION AND PLAN FOR A PRACTICAL MEDICAL REFERENCE:
Principal Diseases of the Interior Valley of North America

The germ of this work was a pamphlet entitled "Notices Concerning Cincinnati," printed for distribution 40 years ago. The greater part of the Interior Valley of North America was at that time a primitive wilderness. Ten years afterward, the author formed the design of preparing a more extended work, on the diseases of the Ohio Valley; but being called to teach, he became interested in medical school which, with the ceaseless labors of medical practice, for the next 20 years, left no time for personal observation, beyond the immediate sphere of his own business.

The object proposed in the following work is to give an account of the causes, symptoms, pathology, and treatment of the principal diseases of an extensive portion of North America—its Interior Valley.... As announced on the title page, it is the design of this work to treat of the diseases of the Caucasian, Indian, and African varieties of our population, in contrast and comparison with each other—the first being the standard to which the other two are brought. For this purpose, no other country presents equal advantages; since, in no other, do we find masses of three varieties of the human race, in permanent juxta-position. There is, moreover, a fourth variety, the Mongolian, represented by the tribes of Esquimaux [Eskimo], whose huts of snow are scattered across the northern extremity of the valley; who subsist on a simpler diet, and live in a lower temperature, than any other known portion of the human race; and, therefore, present, in their habits and physiology, many points of interest, to which he has given such attention as the books of voyages and travels, have enabled him to bestow.

But while the object of this work is to embody facts, drawn, by personal intercourse, from numerous living physicians, or from publications made by them and their predecessors, and to combine the whole with his own observations, he has not been unmindful of the discoveries and improvements in etiology, pathology, and practice, of older and more enlightened countries; but sought, as far as they have become known to him, to amalgamate the foreign with the indigenous, and thus presented to his brethren of the Interior Valley, a book of practice, so full on the diseases in which it treats, as to make it a useful manual for daily reference.

He is obliged to admit, however, that while seeking after knowledge among the physicians of his own country, he could give a little attention to the writings of those who live in other countries. Long journeys of observation, repeated to a large part of several years, with elementary teaching in winter, have much abridged the time for bibliothecal research, and, perhaps, even diminished the taste for that mode of inquiry.

In exploring it (North America—its Interior Valley), for the purpose of collecting facts, the author endeavored to leave behind him all opinions but the single one, that he would observe correctly, must have no theories either to maintain or destroy. To say that he is always been faithful to this rule of observation, would be rash; but he may say, that he has sincerely and earnestly desired, to keep himself under its sway. He may affirm, still further, that it has been his constant aim, to purify from error, the facts he was collecting; and he trusts, therefore, that all the more important be found substantially correct.

Systematic Treatise, Historical, Etiological, and Practical, on the Principal Diseases of the Interior Valley of North America as They Appear in the Caucasian, African, Indian, and Esquimaux Varieties of Its Population. Cincinnati: Winthrop B. Smith & Co., 1850. v–viii.

READER REFLECTION

1. *Do you have an idea for a book? Where did that "germ of a work" begin? Who would benefit (what is your audience)?*
2. *What barriers prevent you from beginning?*
3. *What will be your approach to "gather data"? Fieldwork? Travels for primary observation? Interviews? Reading widely?*
4. *Consider the subjective and objective voices of the work: interpreting the data and presenting facts.*

3.18 INTRODUCING MEDICAL TOPOGRAPHY

The hydrographical map which forms the front piece of this book [*Principal Diseases of the Interior Valley of North America*] seemed indispensable to its plan. The reader will perceive that it is not designed to represent civil and political divisions; but to assist in connecting what is said on medical topography, climate, and the limits imposed by latitude and altitude, on certain diseases, into one system. It was drawn by Major D. P. Whiting, USA, who also drew several of the topographical maps; the remainder and larger part were from the accurate pencil of Captain C. A. Fuller, US civil engineer. They were all executed under the author's inspection, out of the best materials he could command; for a part of which, together with many useful suggestions, he is indebted to the veteran topographical engineer, Col. Stephen H. Long, USA. The engravings are on stone, by a young German artist, Mr. A Wocher of Cincinnati, and will, the author trusts, be found not unworthy of the typographical execution under the supervision of Mr. Charles H. Bronson, whose abilities and taste as a practical printer have overcome many difficulties resulting from the introduction of more than 100 statistical tables and from the absence of the author at the University of Louisville during the past winter while the work was in the press. Finally, the author desires to express his obligations to Messrs. Winthrop B. Smith and Company, for their willingness to turn aside from their ordinary business, and become the publishers of the largest original work which, as yet, has been written and printed in the Interior Valley; thus rendering it in all respects an indigenous production.

Systematic Treatise, Historical, Etiological, and Practical, on the Principal Diseases of the Interior Valley of North America as They Appear in the Caucasian, African, Indian, and Esquimaux Varieties of Its Population. Cincinnati: Winthrop B. Smith & Co., 1850. vii.

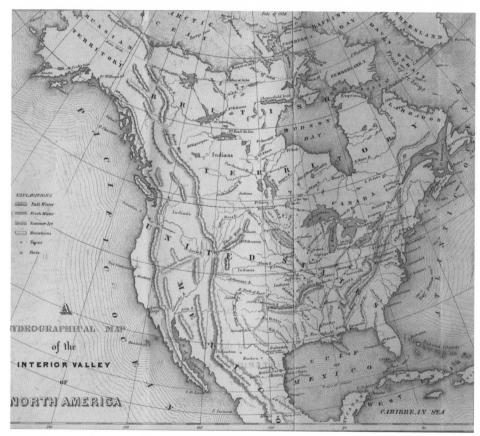

Map of the Interior Valley of North America included in Drake's book *Systematic Treatise on the Principal Diseases of the Interior Valley of North America (1850). Digital copy courtesy of the Henry R. Winkler Center for the History of Health Professions.*

1. *Medical topography is becoming increasing common to reveal patterns of disease. Could this be an effective way to present a story you are seeking to tell in your work?*

2. *Support local and get the best. Drake could have sought out publishers from the east coast but instead supported local artists and printers to do the work. He also sought out the best materials and cartographers he could find. When you need to outsource or tap into expertise on a project do you look locally?*

✖ 3.19 PROPOSING A NEEDED TEXTBOOK IN PATHOLOGY

As far as we know, the first chair of General and Pathological Anatomy instituted in the United States, is that of the new medical department of the Cincinnati College.... Dr. [Samuel] Gross, the professor, a gentleman whose course of studies and mental temperament peculiarly qualify him for the duties of a such a chair, has already made a valuable collection of morbid specimens, which he is augmenting daily. They will be arranged in the College edifice, and at all times open to the inspection of the members of the profession, from whom, in turn, the Doctor will be gratified to receive such specimens of a similar kind, as occasional post mortem examinations may put in their [the examiners'] possession. They should be accompanied with an account of the symptoms under which the patients, from whom they were taken, labored. To fit a specimen for transportation, it should be thoroughly washed with cold water, and then corked or sealed up in a wide mouth bottle, entirely full of strong whiskey or alcohol. Dr. Gross will also be thankful for the specimens taken from brute animals, which should also be accompanied with notices of the fatal symptoms.

"Study of General and Pathological Anatomy." *Western Journal of the Medical and Physical Sciences* 9 (1835): 371–372.

Dr. Drake is engaged in preparing for the press a first book of Pathology; designed, especially for students; and to be comprised in about 450 octavo pages— price three dollars. The views embraced in it will be, substantially, those which he has been accustomed to present, in the introductory part of his course of public lectures, since the year 1825. Their character is well known to many of those who are now practitioners in the Valley of the Mississippi; and they can judge how far his contemplated work will aid them in the difficult task of instructing their students in the rudiments of pathology. He does not anticipate for it a favorable reception in the East of the mountains; but is not without hope that it will attract some share of attention in the West and South; on which he proposes to rely, for the sale of a limited, experimental edition. Unable as yet to find a publisher, he expects to be compelled either to abandon the undertaking or publish it himself. The latter alternative will be adopted, should he find that those for whom the work is particularly intended, are desirous of procuring it.... Should it be produced, he hopes to have it ready for delivery by the first of November; that it may be made the textbook of his lectures on General Pathology, to the students of the Cincinnati College at its next session.

"Elements of Pathology." *Western Journal of the Medical and Physical Sciences* 11 (1838): 642–643.

READER REFLECTION

Note it was not Drake, but instead Dr. Samuel Gross who published Elements of Pathological Anatomy, *2 vols. (Boston: Marsh, 1839), the only comprehensive textbook of pathology in the United States until 1908.*

1. *Producing an innovative work can come from collaboration (here Drake and Gross). Consider sharing an idea with a prospective collaborator who could enhance your project.*
2. *Writers often have ideas for a book that may fill a specific need. Brainstorm such a list of possible books in your field of work.*

3.20 ADVOCACY: THE PURSUIT AND ACQUISITION OF KNOWLEDGE PAYS RICH DIVIDENDS AND IS WORTHY OF SUPPORT

I will indulge the hope, that we shall, at no distant time, more fully perceive and acknowledge the momentous truths, that in a nation organized like ours, private and public prosperity are inseparable. That knowledge is the common basis of both. That efforts to promote it can neither exhaust nor impoverish. That expenditures for its cultivation would not dry up our resources, but, like the exhalations which the earth sends forth, to fall, after a time, in fertilizing showers, would return upon us a rich and replenishing harvest. That periods of great pecuniary embarrassment should not be suffered to diminish these appropriations, as that would inevitably augment the evil. That the greatest number of disasters, both public and private, originate in ignorance, and should not be allowed to perpetuate themselves by fortifying its empire. That under all the vicissitudes and trials of life, after a sincere invocation to Divine Providence, the safest reliance is on the dictates of learning and science; and that in the midst of the widest desolation, our exertions for their benefit should never relax.

An Anniversary Discourse, On the State and Prospects of the Western Museum Society. Cincinnati: Looker, Palmer, and Reynolds, 1820.

READER REFLECTION

1. *Here is an example of Drake's using his powers of the written word to stimulate the reader or hearer to support the growth of learning and science. Why? He argues that an educated public, particularly in the sciences, secures the independence of a nation. Do you agree with this? Is this a sentiment among the people in your community?*

3.21 ADVOCACY: PUBLIC LETTERS IN SUPPORT OF HENRY CLAY FOR PRESIDENT (1824)

Fellow Citizens! The time has now arrived when we should seriously and deeply ponder on the great question [of] who shall be the next President? Heretofore, it might have been proper to listen mainly to the Editors of newspapers, many of whom are intelligent men, if not wise politicians; but in the progress of every national discussion, and on the pendency of every great crisis in the affairs of the Union, it becomes our imperious duty to inquire and think for ourselves. The nation is about to appoint an agent of various powers, many of which, if well defined, are of difficult execution; while others, as the recommendation of new laws, and the nomination of new officers, are entirely discretionary, and at the same time cannot fail to exert much influence on our destinies and happiness.

As an important portion of the American people, it is our duty on this occasion to refer to the situation of the whole, and give our suffrages to no candidate not able and likely to administer the affairs of the Union in such manner as to promote the interests of the majority. At the same time, we cannot promote the interests of the whole, without first considering the interests of all the parts; and as every section of the Union is competent from political knowledge to look after its own immediate concerns, it is correct and necessary for us to do likewise. In fact, people made up as we are can adopt no other plan for their efforts at self-governance. Taking care, then, not to sacrifice the interests of sister states, but to promote them, what is the best policy for us to pursue? On this question no citizen of Ohio or indeed of the West can I apprehend or entertain a doubt. We should promote that system which will bind us to the elder sisters of the republic and promote our internal strength—develop our resources. These ideas may seem trite and commonplace. So much the better.... Believing as I conscientiously do, that no other system of policy can perpetuate the Union, or promote the happiness of the Western States, I should be inconsistent not to introduce them; and not merely introduce them, but to insist that we should dwell on them....

Let us inquire then who among the different distinguished citizens named for the Presidency is most like to administer its government on these principles? Among the candidates for this office, I prefer Mr. Clay.... As it is, the friends of Internal Improvements must rest their hopes upon that gentleman, and happily, all who have studied his character as statesman, will do it with perfect confidence. The traits of that character are too strong, and have been strikingly misunderstood. He has been a public servant for twenty years. But few of the duties assigned him have been performed in an obscure corner of the Republic or a foreign court. His chief scene of action has been the House of Representatives—decidedly the best school for a Statesman this country afford.

Among the numerous actors on that great theatre, he has long been conspicuous as an independent and enlightened patriot; a vigilant sentinel of Republican principles; an eloquent and able advocate of that system of policy by which only this nation can be rendered strong in its resistance to attacks from without or faction within. From the same elevated stage he has, with the eye of a keen and impartial observer, perceived and appreciated the wants and the interests of the various sections of the Union. But it has not been in the political center only that Mr. Clay found opportunities for studying the character and genius of our whole people, and of becoming national in his views. Incredible as it may seem to the city politicians of the Atlantic states, a residence in the Western country is peculiarly calculated to enlarge and liberalize the mind of a statesman. In an emigrant population, like that of the West—presenting endless diversities and combinations—false and contracted views of national character could scarcely be formed or cherished.... An inhabitant of the West is, therefore, of necessity more national than one of the East or the South, because the East and the South have united to form the West.

"The Presidency I & II." *Liberty Hall & Cincinnati Gazette*, April 20 and 27, 1824.

1. *Identify an area that you are passionate about that needs reform or change. Or consider a political candidate that you support. Write a letter of advocacy to the appropriate audience.*

⬛ 3.22 ADVOCACY: CALLING OUT THE NEED FOR EDUCATIONAL REFORM

During the last 30 years I have become acquainted with the literary and professional ignorance of so many students and physicians, in and of various parts of the union, that I cannot be mistaken in asserting, that the majority of the profession in America are deficient in common school learning. If such be the fact, it should not be considered libelous to publish it, especially when done by one who claims no exemption from the imperfections which he deplores. So long as we "measure ourselves by ourselves and compare ourselves among ourselves" we are not likely either to perceive or supply our defects. There can be no true reformation without a consciousness of its necessity; and if these remarks and should contribute, but in the slightest degree, to excite it, I shall submit cheerfully to the odium which they may bring upon me, from those who find determination more convenient than improvement.

But is the education which our common schools confer, a sufficient preparation for the study of medicine? It certainly is not....

The United States are, perhaps, the only civilized country in modern times, where it has been seriously doubted whether the languages and literature of the ancients should make a part of the studies of professional man. Of the various causes which have combined to suggest this question, one of the most operative is the spirit of liberal inquiry, which originated, and is cherished by, our free institutions. No people are so unshackled by prejudices and precedents; none so excursive; none so experimental, as the American. If they do not "try all things, and hold fast to that which is good," they try many, and are strongly disposed to fix upon something new....

...It would be in vain to hope, that a due respect for the learned languages, or even a conviction of their utility, could survive...and hence we find, that in the United States, a want of acquaintance with them, has been no serious obstacle to the attainment of high relative distribution, in any of the pursuits of society.... A perception of their value appears to be returning.... Meanwhile, it is the duty of those who can exercise any control over public sentiment in this respect, to exert themselves; and, if all who are interested in the dignity of the medical profession, could be brought to unite their efforts in favor of a more classical preparation of young men designed for study, it cannot be doubted, that much might be accomplished, even in a single generation.

"Selection and Preparatory Education of Pupils." In *Practical Essays on Medical Education and the Medical Profession in the United States.* Cincinnati: Roff & Young, 1832. 12–14,15.

READER REFLECTION

1. *Consider the quality of training in your field or career. What is the state of your profession, and where are the gaps in preparation and education? What could be improved? Draft a position statement.*
2. *What needs reform in your profession? What could be written to guide or stimulate reform?*
3. *Consider the benefits of studying the works and lives of those individuals in your field from previous generations.*

✖ 3.23 ADVOCACY: THE NEED FOR REFORM OF MEDICAL EDUCATION

The consequences of this deficiency of talent in the profession are of serious import to the science and to the people at large. It is unquestionably one of the causes which retard the progress of discovery and improvement. Of the thousands who annually go forth with diplomas or licenses, or without either, to engage in the practical duties of the profession, very few ever contribute a single new fact to its archives, or communicate an impulse to the minutest wheel in its complicated machinery. Acting on the precepts of others they may, it is true, do some good, but they also do much harm; while to the great work of revising and correcting the principles of science they are of course utterly incompetent.

But this incompetency is not the effect of inferior talents only; it results, perhaps, in an equal degree from want of education and mental discipline. Although medicine is ranked with the *learned* professions not a few of its professors are deficient in learning. This is the case not only in the Western states where for obvious reasons it might be expected; but in almost every part of the union with the exception of our large cities. Writing as I do for practical effect and to promote reform I am constrained to say the profession abounds in students and practitioners who are radically defective in spelling, grammar, etymology, descriptive geography, arithmetic, and I might add, book-keeping.... Were this confined to unauthorized members of the profession it would be an affair of little magnitude, but extending to many of the graduates of all our Universities, it calls for unreserved exposure and unqualified reprehension.

"Selection and Preparatory Education of Pupils." In *Practical Essays on Medical Education and the Medical Profession in the United States*. Cincinnati: Roff & Young, 1832. 11–12.

READER REFLECTION

1. *Taking an unpopular stand or exposing falsehood takes courage and can make enemies. What motivates a person to take this on in the face of opposition?*

2. *Calling for reform is a call to improve. Consider if continuous improvement is or should be part of your organization.*

3. *How can you promote the goal for all physicians to be practicing scientists and staying intellectually curious?*

⊠ 3.24 DEFENSE AFTER DISMISSAL FROM THE MEDICAL COLLEGE OF OHIO

The following narrative relates chiefly to the writer himself.... He has not written for the inhabitants of Cincinnati, merely—who are in general already acquainted with the events of which he treats; but for the people of the State—to whom, from the interest they have manifested towards the Medical College, it is due to give a statement of the causes which have reduced it from five to two professors;—and for the Western public at large,—to whom it is equally due, to be made acquainted with the character of the remaining incumbents.

He was, in truth, reluctant to write at all; and has therefore suffered nearly two months to elapse, from the close of the drama which he describes, in hopes of being able to produce a state of things that would render a resort to the press unnecessary for the vindication of his character.... *The time and reputation of a professional man are his capital....* Whether by this resort he will be found to have accomplished the object in view, remains to be seen. He cannot but be sensible, that the very means of defense which he has been compelled to employ, may possibly stir up the wrath of his standing enemies; but at this late period, he is not to be deterred or startled by such an apprehension. He has followed as the subject led; and will rest satisfied, if in giving the history of a corrupt and complicated transaction, he shall be found to have said nothing to forfeit the respect of his friends or the confidence of the public....

Three charges have been often made against me, to which I propose to respond. I will consider them separately.

1. That among my medical brethren I am quarrelsome. The whole of my public controversies with any of the medical men, of this or any other place, have been since the year 1818; the time when I formed and expressed the design of instituting a medical school; and they have all grown directly or indirectly out of that design. From that date, in ambush or open day, they have waged upon me a predatory war; and when I have defended either the object or myself, they have with one voice exclaimed—"What an awful quarrelsome man! How dreadful broilsome he is! No soul lives in harmonious concord with him! But for him we should be as one might say, a body of brethren. We have tried by every art not to irritate him, until we are really discouraged, and cannot do anything more! He is so pugnacious, that he contends with a dozen of us at once; and until society will frown him into due submissiveness, or what would suit our interests better, drive him into banishment, they cannot expect to enjoy the sweets of peaceful tranquility!"

To this effect have been the pacific and pathetic vociferations of my humble aggressors, whenever I was driven into resistance, and happened to make reprisals upon them; and by such appeals they have expected to perform what there was no hope accomplishing in any other way. Like certain heroes of the *Dunciad* [mock heroic poem by Alexander Pope] they have great faith in the power of noise; and it must be allowed, that of all the torrents that can be formed in society against an individual, no one is more difficult to stem than a clamor. Whether that which they have labored to raise, can be made strong enough to sweep me away, time only can determine.

2. That I have cultivated other branches of science than my profession.

I should feel proud to plead guilty to this charge without qualification. It is true that I believe, in common with many other physicians, that the science of medicine consists of something more than a collection of infallible receipts; that it is indeed a wide spreading branch of the great stock of human knowledge; and that in pursuing its ramifications we are often drawn into a temporary study of the objects with which they are entwined—I have moreover perceived, that our country abounds in the unopened and ample stores of nature's productions, and have delivered an elementary course of lecture on Botany, and another on Mineralogy, with the sole view of inspiring my young countryman with a taste of those sciences; but even when thus employed—while held in transient captivity within their magic circles—I have never forgotten that they are but the auxiliary organs

LEAVING A LEGACY

of the profession, and entitled only to the homage of a secondary devotion. The scientific world would be amused to learn, that such a charge has been brought against a man, who has contributed little more to their journals, than his accusers, who have contributed nothing.

I shall dismiss this allegation, and proceed to the last.

3. That I am ambitious.

The objects of my ambition have been a Public Library—a School of Literature and the Arts for the promotion of useful knowledge—a Lancaster Seminary, with a superadded Grammar School, and a College for classical education, supervening upon this—a Museum, in which lectures on the curious production of nature and art might be delivered—a Medical College—a Public Hospital and Lunatic Asylum for the state. All of these have been originated with the last 10 years; and each of them I have had the honor, with a little band of ardent and munificent spirits, to be a laborer. The difficulties we have had to encounter, have been neither new nor feeble. As old ones have been vanquished new ones have appeared; and to borrow a metaphor, like the one traveller ascending the Alps, we have only surmounted one, to be presented with another....

I was personally desirous of seeing a liberal and permanent medical school established in Cincinnati; the town of all others in the western country which has the greatest number of natural advantages for such an institution....

The labors of this place will not, however, be ultimately unproductive. In the cycle of changes an auspicious hour will sooner or later arrive, when the Medical College, and any of our other institutions which appear to be now prostrate, may be revived and made to shed upon the society the fruits, which, in a flourishing condition, they cannot fail to produce. But before this can take place, the community become more united; their countenance must be withdrawn from those who, out of selfish motives, array themselves in opposition; the labor and the contribution must not be expected from a few; nor must it be a reproach to those who dedicate themselves to this services, that they are ambitious.

A Narrative of the Rise and Fall of the Medical College of Ohio. Cincinnati: Looker & Reynolds, Printers, 1822. v, vi, 36–40.

Reader Reflection

1. *Think of a time when your character or reputation was under attack. How did you respond? Would you have done anything different looking back on that time?*

2. *Don't be surprised of opposition when seeking to start something new. Discuss: Part of a person's legacy is in surmounting obstacles.*

3.25 Use of Humor: A Novel Site for Smallpox Vaccination

Why does not some one get out a patent for preventing the small pox by vaccinating on the nose, instead of the arm? It might be averred, that it would not, then, be necessary to repeat the operation every seven years; or oftener, when a man moved from one town to another. Such vaccinations would be as effective as those in the arm, and could be referred to and published—not as testimony in favor of the *Cow-pock*, but in favor of inserting it in the end of the snout. Thus, in a short time, we should find half the community—(we mean half in point of numbers) turning up their noses at their incredulous and bigoted brethren, who might prefer to have the carbuncle on their arms.

"The People's Doctors; a Review by 'The People's Friend.'{hrs}" *Western Journal of the Medical and Physical Sciences* 3 (1829): 393–420, 455–462.

Reader Reflection

1. *Try using humor to communicate a point.*

3.26 Writing to Combat Quackery: "The People's Doctors"

"They shall have mysteries—aye precious stuff
"For knaves thrive by—mysteries enough;
"Dark tangled doctrines, dark as fraud can weave,
"Which simple votaries shall on trust receive,
"While craftier feign belief, till they believe."

Superstition, says [William?] Robertson, the celebrated historian of America, "was originally engrafted on medicine, not on religion." However this may be, no one conversant with "poor human nature," can be unapprised of the close companionship which has always subsisted between them. In savage life, a belief in the healing efficacy of charms and incantations is so universal, as to leave no doubt that a principle of superstition is inherent in the human mind. It belongs, therefore, to man in every situation; though in civilized life its manifestations are comparably few and feeble, for it is the tendency of all good education to limit its operations. Hence the most enlightened minds, display the least propensity for the marvelous; but how can the intellect of the whole nation be cultivated on all subjects? This was never yet done, and we are sorry to add, never can be done. In despite of every exertion to illuminate the mass, many dark and impenetrable spots will remain; so that society, in its best composition, must continue to display enough credulity to render it ridiculous. From the depths of ignorance, with its overshadowing superstitions,—when the hopes of the sick rest upon spells and coscinomancy [a form of divination],—the first step taken, is to blend with these supernatural, a variety of natural means, resting the efficacy of the latter, on the occult influence of the former. The next advance leaves the mummeries of the sorcerer behind; but clings to amulets, seventh-sons, "yarb-doctors," and vagabonds.

This brings us to our own age—than which, with all our boasted elevation in learning and philosophy, no other has ever presented a greater variety of barefaced and abominable quackeries. To eradicate them would be more difficult than to root out the sour dock and the Canada thistle of our fields, while the soil continues to favor their reproduction. Planted in the ignorance of the multitude, warmed by its credulity, and cherished by their artful and unblushing authors, these imposters are fixed upon us, as the "poison oak" encircles the trunk of the noble tree, whose name it has prostituted. True it is, they are not always the same. The stupidest intellect at last comes to perceive their absurdity, and throws them off; but the imposters— "New edge their dullness and new bronze their face"—and speedily invent fresh draughts for the gaping and thirsty populace.

When one of these quackeries is inoculated into a community, nothing can arrest its spread, or limit its duration. Every dog has its day, and so has every nostrum. The gulping is universal; not extending, it is true, to every individual, but all classes. The propensity to be cheated is not confined to men or women, the old or young, the poor or rich, the unlearned, or (we are sorry to add) the learned; but displays its workings in the weak-minded and credulous of all. Like the small pox it prevails till all the susceptible are infected, and have gone through the disease. A moment of common sense may, perhaps, succeed to the period of suffering; as natural fools have sometimes spoken well from the shock of a violent blow. The desire to be cheated, however, returns apace; but not earlier than the desire to cheat—

> "Then thick as locusts dark'ning all the ground,
> "A tribe, with herbs and roots fantastic crown'd,
> "All with some wond'rous gift approach the people,
>   "—Lobelia, pulmel, and steam kettle."

But it is time to enter on the review of the important works which lie before us.

Of these books, the first is by *doctor* [Samuel] Thomson, who has favored the public [with] *New Guide to Health; or, Botanic Family Physician* [Columbus: Horton Howard, 1828] "containing a complete system of practice upon a plan entirely new; with descriptions of the vegetables made use of, and directions for preparing and administering them to cure disease."

The first 30 pages are composed of interlarded sketches, of the author's birth, labors, and persecutions; of warnings to the good people against the "regular faculty," and of his system of physiology, pathology, and therapeuticks....

The following extract will no doubt impart much consolation and quiet of conscience, to some of the regular faculty.

> "It is true that the study of anatomy, or structure of the human body and of the whole animal economy, is pleasing and useful; nor is there any objection to this, however minute and critical, it is not to know the neglect of first great principles, and the weightier matters of knowledge. But it is no more necessary to mankind at large, to qualify them to administer relief from pain and sickness, than to cook in preparing food to satisfy hunger and nourishing the body. There is one general cause of hunger and one general supply of food; one general cause of disease and one general remedy. One can be satisfied, the other removed, by an infinite variety of articles, best adapted to those different purposes—That medicine, therefore, will open obstruction, promote perspiration, and restore digestion, is suited to

every patient, whatever form the disease assumes, and is universally applicable."

But it is time to enter the steam bath. Here the doctor is quite at home; and when at home does least harm to his patients.

"Steaming is a very important branch of my system of practice, which would in many cases without it, be insufficient to effect a cure. It is of great importance in many cases considered by the medical faculty as desperate; and they would be so under my mode of treatment, if it were not for this manner of applying heat to the body, for the purpose of reanimating the system and aiding nature in restoring health. I had but little knowledge of medicine, when through necessity, I discovered the use of steaming, to add heat of life to the decaying spark; and with it I was enabled, by administering such vegetable preparations as I then had knowledge of, to effect a cure in cases where regular practitioners had given them over.

The method adopted by me, and which has always answered the desired object, is as follows—Take several stones of different sizes and put them in the fire till red hot, then take the smallest first, and put on of them into a pan or kettle of hot water, and with the stone about half immersed—the patient must be undressed and a blanket about him so as to shield his whole body from the air, and then place him over the steam. Change the stones as often as they grow cool, so as to keep up a lively steam, and keep them over it; if they are faint throw a little cold water on the face and stomach, which will let down the outward heat and restore strength—after they have been over the steam long enough, which will generally be about 15 or 20 minutes they must be washed all over with cold water or spirits and put in bed, or may be dressed, as the circumstances of the case shall permit."

...The originality of this method certainly entitled it to a patent.

It is marvelous that intelligent men should not open their eyes to the real character of this quackery. It presents us with the very first example on record, of a patent for the practice of medicine. The profits of the patent right are in proportion to the number of individual patents, each $20, which can be sold.... No education is necessary to qualify [to use this method in] practice, except enough to read Thomson's directions; they are not, in any case, responsible for the result, and have no professional character to support.

By the light of these facts no one can fail to perceive, what an immense influence is brought to bear upon the community in favor of this patent.... Being... disseminated by his patent, we cannot refrain from adding, that it is discreditable to our age and nation, that such patents should ever be issued. *Indeed the whole practice of the government on this point is radically wrong, and should not be reformed, but renounced.* No modification of it could confer on society so great a benefit as its total abolition.

"The People's Doctors; a Review by 'The People's Friend.'{hrs}" *Western Journal of the Medical and Physical Sciences* 3 (1829): 393–420, 455–462.

READER REFLECTION

1. *What books are current that include fantastic, untested claims that mislead many?*
2. *Try writing a satirical essay in review of a common form of quackery.*

✠ 3.27 POETRY: "MY MOTHER"
On her 70th Birthday-September 20th, 1831

Who toiled by day and sunk to rest
With me upon her wearied breast
And hushed my cries and called me "bless'd"?
My Mother

As on the grass I crept and laugh'd
And furious mad-dog near me passed
Who shrieked and frantic, stood aghast?
My Mother

When first I clamber'd o'er the sill,
And totter'd onward to the mill,
Who brought me back against my will?
                    My Mother

When duty bid, who sad forsook
Her native plains and dear Greenbrook
And westward cast an anxious look?
                    My Mother

Who up the mountains rocky side
Each act of pleasing family tried
When I would neither walk nor ride?
                    My Mother

Who reach'd the dark deep western wood
Embark'd on bright Ohio's flood,
And timid sought the "Land of blood"?
                    My Mother

Who in the ark which floated on
Through solitudes to her unknown,
Hath watch upon her heedless son?

                    My Mother

Who in the sun's red beams afar,
Or in the brilliant setting star,
Beheld the savage fires of war?
                    My Mother

Who heard dismay'd from either shore
The hidden cataracts distant roar
Flout in the echo of the oar?
                    My Mother

Who startled in her troubled dream,
As o'er the surface of the stream,
The panther sent his hideous scream?
                    My Mother

Who in each fallen floating tree
Through midnight mists would trembling see
The pirogue of the enemy?
My Mother

Who shudder'd when the Indian's yell
Rose, horrid, from the gloomy dell,
And told the bleeding infant's knell?
My Mother

Who in a floorless cabin slept,
As round her bed the lizards crept?
Or o'er her babies watch'd and wept?
My Mother

Who as she left her sleepless bed,
The silent tear of anguish shed,
To hear me cry in vain for bread?
My Mother

Who saw in dreams around her stand
The comforts of her native land
And grasp'd but work'd with empty hand?
My Mother

Who in my dinner basket plac'd
"Old Dilworth" back'd with rags and paste
And bid me to school house haste?
My Mother

Who dress'd me in my Sunday clothes
And grac'd my bosom with a rose,
And made me outward turn my toes?
My Mother

Who brought in doors the freezing lamb,
And bade Sis warm it near the jamb,
While I spread husks around its dam?
My Mother

Who anxious watch'd the evening star
And heard with joy the falling bar,
When I return'd from mill, afar?
                                    My Mother

Who listen'd for the horse's tramp,
At dead of night when from the camp,
We brought the maple sugar damp?
                                    My Mother

Who quickly spread the frugal meal,
And supper o'er prepar'd to kneel,
And join in pray'r with faith and zeal?
                                    My Mother

The parting came as years roll'd on,
Who now embrac'd her youthful son,
And bid him go, then mourn'd him gone?
                                    My Mother

Now that disease and age have shed
Their baleful influence on thy head,
Look to thy God and fear no dread,
                                    My Mother

Verse Album of Daniel Drake, 1830–1836. Emmet Field Horine Papers (67M149), 1788–1863, Box 20, Folder 1. King Library, University of Kentucky Special Collections.

3.28 POETRY: "HYMN FOR MY MOTHER'S FUNERAL, NOVEMBER 10TH 1831"

When humble Christians feel the blow,
And sink resigned on Jesus's breast,
We should not mourn to see them go
And mingle, joyful with the bless'd.

No more they drink the bitter draught
Of disappointment, pain and grief;
On every sigh no longer waft
A pray'r for mercy and relief.

Their troubled dream of life is o'er,
No more by storms can they be driven,
They rest upon the happy shore—
Behind them Earth, before them Heaven.

Behold that quiet smiling face!
It speaks of joys beyond the tomb,
Of Jesus's love and pardoning grace,
And, with the Savior, bids us come.

There let us mourn not for the dead,
But humbly lift the chast'ning rod,
Look up to him who for us bled,
And live prepared to meet our God.

Verse Album of Daniel Drake, 1830–1836. Emmet Field Horine Papers (67M149), 1788–1863, Box 20, Folder 1. King Library, University of Kentucky Special Collections.

✠ 3.29 PRIVATE JOURNAL: REFLECTING ON MARITAL LOVE AFTER MY WIFE'S DEATH

Our marriage was from love; our love from mutual respect and esteem. It rested on no considerations of family or fortune, was excited and inflamed by no arts or affection. It was spontaneous sentiment in both souls, and rose simultaneously.

I was twenty-two, she twenty. In person she was of middle stature or rather less, with a comely though not beautiful form, but erect, elastic, and dignified; in countenance animated, forceful, expressive; free from affected looks and gestures; inclining to an aspect of honest and native pride. The great charm of her presence was simplicity. Her appearance and manner exhibited not less *naiveté* than her conversation. This was always marked by good sense and good feeling. Her opportunities of acquiring knowledge, particularly scholastic learning, had been limited; but her observation of those about her and of society was acute and discriminating. She saw with accuracy and judged with correctness. She expressed herself with the modesty which pervaded all her actions. In mixed circles she was silent. To her immediate friends and associates only she disclosed the intrinsic beauties of her soul. In regard to marriage her great maxim was, to marry for love, and to love from manifestations of character.

Our courtship was not coy, nor formal, nor protracted. My desires and designs were made known to her guardian aunt, Mrs. Colonel Jared Mansfield; before they had been, in words, communicated to herself. They were approved by her to whom they were addressed; and nature had already assured me they would be approved by her who was their object. A few interviews brought us to a full understanding, almost independently of the use of words. We conversed on the objections which each might find in the other; and while contemplating the obstacles to a union, our spirits imperceptibly commingled into one. Perfect reciprocal confidence arose before we were conscious of perfect love; and ere the marriage rites were performed, our fortunes and fates were indissolubly united and ours souls consecrated to each other.

"Emotions, Reflections, and Anticipations" [1826 or 1827]. In *Pioneer Life in Kentucky: A Series of Reminiscential Letters from Daniel Drake, M.D., of Cincinnati to His Children,* edited by Charles D. Drake. Cincinnati: Robert Clarke & Co., 1870. xiv.

Reader Reflection

1. *Discuss the foundation of marriage based on mutual respect, esteem for the other person, reciprocal confidence, and consecration to the other. What legacy might such a marriage leave to the children?*
2. *If married how would you write about your relationship? Compare and contrast your view with the experience of Daniel and Harriet Drake.*

3.30 Poetry: "The Lover's Winter Visit"

Written on my 25th Wedding day–December 22nd, 1832

December blew his frosty breath
And wept the beauteous vale in death.

The whisp'ring zephyr caused to blow
The rippling brooks forgot to glow
The water fall and latt'ring mill,
Awake no echoes on the hill.
The wither'd rose leaves fall'n and dead
Beneath the snow, no fragrance shed;
The evening star casts forth no gleam
To sparkle joyous on the stream;
No silent lightings flash'd at even,
Nor rising moon shone light in Heav'n.
No firefly shed her summer glow
In mellow splendors on the snow;
The whippoorwill, her vesper lay
No longer caroled on the way;
No noisy katydid now play'd
The musing traveler serenade.

But though the chill and dreary gloom
Like wailing voices from the tomb
If the past year, the northern breeze
Swept dismal o'er the leafless trees
It caus'd the snow drift, where the flow'r
Late bloom'd beneath the past leav'r
And in the darkness of that night
Fall but the faint and yellow light
Which through the cabin's open seams
Came dimly forth in flick'ring streams.

Now who is he these gleams disclose
Calm struggling through those drifting snows?
Whose fiery steed the pierce wind's wrath
Braves snorting on the treacherous path?
A sanguine youth with flaxen hair,
And brow of thought slight bent with care,
A son of nature more than art,
Of rustic mien but with a heart

To time so faithful and so warm
He's boldly fac'd the driving storm
A joyous youth with hopes unblighted
His holy vows not scorn'd or slight'd;
Whose fancy rear'd the home of love,
And fondly plac'd it far above
All storms of sorrow and distress
The home of peace and happiness.

And who is she that fires his soul
As round his head the tempest howl?
The living star whose gentle say
Could guide him on the dangerous way?
The loveliest maiden of the vale,
The fairest flower of Harriet-dale.
The modest eye of hazel hue
Disclosed e'en to the passing view
Truth, firmness, feeling, innocence
Bright thoughts and deep intelligence.
Keen soul was pure as winter's snow
And warm as summer's sunniest glow.
When moving through the mingled crowd
Her lofty bearing spoke her proud.
For pride and patience own'd her pow'r
Ere yet her brow began to low'r
But when her kindling spirit breath'd
On those she lov'd or those who griev'd
Joy felt, his quicken'd pulses leap
And sorrow e'en forgot to weep.

Before the hospitable fire
Pensive she sat in deep desire,
That he might safely quickly come
Or hop'd he had not quit his home,
That ruthless night. Then down the vale
Her sighs went floating on the gale

To fall upon her lover's ear,
And till that she who sigh'd was near;
And so they did or might have done
For now his prize was nearly won
Before she heav'd a second sigh
The faithful watchdog told him nigh
And as another moment flew,
He burst enraptur'd on her view
Smiling he banish'd love's alarms
And clasp'd her in his shiv'ring arms.

A tear and deep emotion plow'd
Slow down her grinning cheek and glow'd
Like dew-drop on the blushing rose
When morn his joyful radiance throws:
That tear which left its fount in sadness
Fell on his throbbing breast in gladness
Thus high amidst the brooding storm,
The flakes of snow have birth and form
But as they reach the opening flowers
Dissolve and fall in April showers.

Verse Album of Daniel Drake, 1830–1836. Emmet Field Horine Papers (67M149), 1788–1863, Box 20, Folder 1. King Library, University of Kentucky Special Collections.

✠ 3.31 POETRY: "HYMN"

Written for the fifth anniversary commemoration [of his wife's death] Sunday Oct 3rd 1830—the 1st being Friday

In Autumn when the rustling leaf
Speaks to the heart and wakes our grief,
We come in evening's quiet hours
To strew thy grave with fading flowers.

To

Harriet Echo

—

My babe! Echo of her I lov'd —
Young joyous thing, by trifles mov'd! —
You claim, — to deck your winter bow'r, —
This half-blown, frozen, pale white flow'r,
Not sown nor watered by the Muses
Like gifted poets fragrant posies; —
—But since to you it seems so fair,
Accept it, with a father's prayer.
△△.

Cin. Feb. 6ᵗʰ 1830.

A hand-written poem of Daniel Drake to his daughter, Harriett Echo Drake, included in *Verse Album of Daniel Drake, 1830–1836. Photo by the author. Courtesy of the University of Kentucky Libraries.*

The simple stone, which shields thy form
From summer's sun and winter's storm
We polish o'er each spot efface
And bind with willow boughs and grass.

Thy seraph voice, lamented shade
Floats mildly in the tranquil air
Accept the homage we have paid
And bids us all for Heaven prepare.

Verse Album of Daniel Drake, 1830–1836. Emmet Field Horine Papers (67M149), 1788–1863, Box 20, Folder 1. King Library, University of Kentucky Special Collections.

▨ 3.32 POETRY: "FUNERAL HYMN FOR THE SIXTH ANNIVERSARY OF HIS WIFE'S DEATH"

October 1st, 1831

Inscribed affectionately to my only son, Charles Daniel

Ye clouds that veil the setting sun
Dye not your robes in red;
Thou chaste and beauteous rising moon
Thy mildest radiance sheds—

Ye stars that give the vault of Heaven
Shine mellow as ye pass;
Ye falling dews of early even'
Rest, balmy on this grass.

Ye fitful zephyrs as ye rise
And win your way along
Breathe softly out your deepest sighs
And wail your gloomiest song:

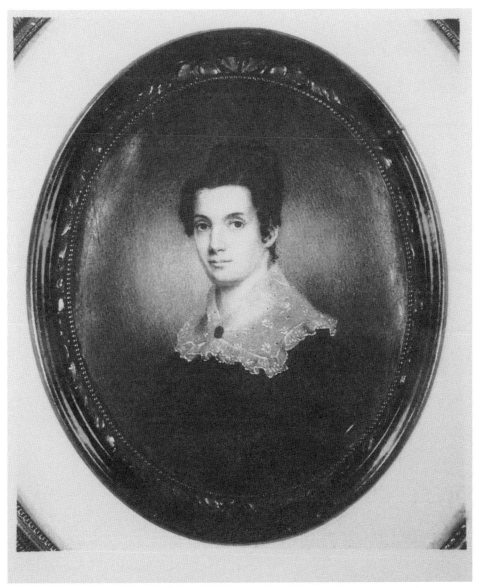

Harriet Sisson Drake, the wife of Daniel Drake, who died September 30, 1825, age thirty-seven. Emmet Field Horine Papers, King Library, the University of Kentucky Libraries Special Collections. *Courtesy of the University of Kentucky Libraries. Photo by the author.*

Thou lonely widowed bird of night;
As on this sacred stone
Thou may'st in wand'rings chance to light,
Pour forth thy saddest means:—

Ye giddy throng who laughing stray
Where notes of grief resound
And mock the funeral vesper lay
Tread not this holy ground;—

For here my sainted Harriet lies,
I saw her hallow'd form
Deep laid below no more to rise,
Before the judgment morn.

Verse Album of Daniel Drake, 1830–1836. Emmet Field Horine Papers (67M149), 1788–1863, Box 20, Folder 1. King Library, University of Kentucky Special Collections.

READER REFLECTION

1. *Poetry is another genre for expressing yourself. For Drake most of his poetry was about people closest to him—his wife, mother, or children. Consider expressing your thoughts of those closest to you in verse.*

2. *Take a moment to reflect on your relationship with your spouse and capture your feelings in verse. What message would that communicate to your spouse? Your children?*

3.33 LETTERS: REMEMBERING THOSE WE HAVE LOST

In many of the labors I have described, and many more with which I cannot find it in my heart to trouble you, my sweet and gentle sister Lizzy was my companion and assistant. I never knew a kinder-hearted child, one more ready and bent on dividing every good thing, and as far as I can now judge, I never loved a human being more tenderly. My very first memory was of her, and her death, while my patient, just thirty years afterward, was a sad affliction.

Our ages were too near for me to be her nurse, but my early remembrances disclose to me, that as soon as she was old enough to be amused, I was employed in that duty, and that as she advanced, I took an out-door charge of her. Subsequently we were employed in common, rocking the cradle, carrying about, tending and taking care of the four younger children, while mother was at work. In this way I became quite a nurse, and to it may ascribe some of my traits of character in after life, which have been sources of both pleasure and profit. I like the society of little children, and their amusements around me excite and interest me, even when I do not observe them. I love to hear their voices, their young laughter cheers me, and their crying, if not from real grief, gives me little disturbance of thought or feeling. Above all, I am delighted to see them aim at becoming members of an older circle, attentive to what is said, and anxious to ask a question or put in a word. After saying this, you will not be surprised when I tell you that I have read many an hour with your husband and his sisters in my arms, often walking with them, and sometimes singing to keep them quiet, while their mother, in our poverty, like my own, was at work in the kitchen or the chamber, alone, or with some miserable servant, such as Cincinnati had, when the soft fibers of my younger heart were interwoven, not tangled, with those of that lovely and beloved woman, so long my devoted companion in the care and troubles of the enjoyment of life.

"Letter to his daughter-in-law." In *Pioneer Life in Kentucky: A Series of Reminiscential Letters from Daniel Drake, M.D., of Cincinnati to His Children*. Edited by Charles D. Drake. Cincinnati: Robert Clark & Co., 1870. 103–104.

READER REFLECTION

1. *In his early sixties Drake recorded some of his early life experiences for his children. Look back and tell your children your story. What would you want to pass on to them?*
2. *What stories of family members now dead would you like to share with your children?*

🏵 3.34 LETTERS: THE REALITY OF DEATH

When I was on the old farm in the spring of 1845, I went to the spot of my first achievement. The slope and jutting rocks were there, but no vestige of living nature remained. Evan a great honey-locust stump, which had stood in my way, had decayed and disappeared. Thus men, and animals, and trees—all that have life—yield to the destroyer, while the mineral features of the earth remain almost unchanged. The fig trees of Judea are no more; but the natural cavern, from which the Savior called forth Lazarus, was. The temple of Solomon has crumbled into dust; but Lebanon, which supplied the cedars which adorned it, still rises in unaltered grandeur. With these evidences before us of the certain destruction of everything which has life, how cheering and glorious is the hope that He who said, "Lazarus, come forth," will, in His own time, call on all who trust in Him to leave the tomb and be with Him.

Pioneer Life in Kentucky: A Series of Reminiscential Letters from Daniel Drake, M.D., of Cincinnati to His Children. Edited by Charles D. Drake. Cincinnati: Robert Clark & Co., 1870. 67–68.

READER REFLECTION

1. *In writing to his children, Drake reminded them of the certainty of death and decay, but also of hope! If you were to communicate your thoughts on death what would you say to your children?*

Educator

"An Eminent Teacher of the Medical Art"

"To be a teacher in his own profession, he thought to be his peculiar gift; nor did he confine himself to that only; he sought the society of clergymen, of professors, teachers, in fine, of all who by teaching sought to improve and regenerate the race."

—Edward D. Mansfield, *Memoirs of the Life and Services of Daniel Drake, M.D.*

4.1   *Beginning as a Teacher*

4.2   *Choosing a Good Teacher*

4.3   *Specific Teaching Methods for Preceptors*

4.4   *Using Experiments and Demonstrations to Teach*

4.5   *Length of Terms and Limitations of Learning from Lectures*

4.6   *Advice for Effective Lecturing*

4.7   *Have Learners Take Notes*

4.8   *Inspire the Love of Learning*

4.9   *Cultivate and Improve the Faculty of Observation*

4.10   *Recognize What Capacities Students Need for a Medical Career*

4.11   *The Cardinal Virtues of a Student*

4.12   *Appreciate the Value of Latin and Greek Languages and Knowledge of the Ancient Texts*

4.13   *Stages to Professional Excellence*

4.14   *Train for Frequent Interruptions*

4.15   *Manage the Day*

4.16   *Take Care of Yourself during Your Student Days*

4.17   *Set Aside Time to Develop Your Character*

4.18   *Acquire the Habit of Managing Your Money and Lifestyle Well*

4.19   *Get a Liberal Arts Education with a Daily Habit*

4.20   *Recognize How Other Fields of Learning Can Inform and Assist Your Work*

4.21   *Principles for Learning and Building a Foundation for Your Profession*

4.22   *Consider the Best Setting for Learning Specific Types of Knowledge*

4.23   *Training for a Special Area: Learning Surgery*

4.24   *Diagnosis Is Learned at the Bedside*

4.25   *Know the Leading Edge of Learning*

4.26   *How to Learn in Practice*

4.27   *Stages of Mastery: Many Fields Have Complex Problems to Solve*

4.28   *Stages of Mastery: The Physician as Scientist, Philosopher, Scholar, and Artist*

4.29   *Lifelong Learning*

Chapter Four

— *Drake was a leader among educators in Ohio and Kentucky. In 1817, he was a faculty member of the first medical institution west of the Allegheny Mountains, the Medical College of Lexington.*

— *As the first president of the Medical College of Ohio in 1819, he remains a prominent figure in the history of the city of Cincinnati and its university.*

— *Drake held professorships in a number of medical subjects, including clinical medicine, theory of practice, botany and materia medica, and pathology, reflecting his broad interests, expertise, and devotion to his students' medical education.*

◪ AUTHOR INTRODUCTION

One of Drake's core strengths was a thirst for learning. This strength began to manifest itself very early in his life. His experiences in Philadelphia at the University of Pennsylvania Medical School introduced him to the leading medical educators of his day and provided examples of effective teaching of medicine. But his appreciation of the value of education was much broader than medicine. He understood the critical importance of education as a cornerstone of a democracy, and as a consequence he was keenly interested in advancing education and the development of teachers. At age twenty-nine he was involved in the creation of the Cincinnati Lancaster Seminary, a system of public education that opened in April 1815. He served as secretary of the board of trustees and assisted in raising money for building and operating the school. It was highly successful and in 1819 merged with the newly chartered Cincinnati College (the forerunner of the University of Cincinnati). Subsequently, in 1832 with the public school movement still in its infancy, Drake became involved in the Western Literary Institute and the College of Professional Teachers, an organization of teachers primarily from Cincinnati, and also interested teachers from the surrounding region. In this group Drake spoke out in support of establishing public schools and compulsory education of children.

Drake revealed he was an innovative, visionary, and remarkably practical educator in many ways. He recognized that to educate students, it was first necessary to train and equip the teachers. In assembling faculty for schools he sought out the best teachers he could find and set high standards. He saw the educational gaps in students entering medical schools and realized to train better doctors, the students needed better education prior to medical school. He also saw the gaps in medical education between the medical school and the apprenticeship model and offered practical solutions to address these gaps. He was learner-centric. One example of this was recognizing that the best way to learn specific clinical skills such as diagnosis, surgery, or obstetrics was to teach these subjects in the hospital at the bedside or operating room and not in lecture halls, as was common in medical schools across the country. Drake called for broader system reforms, and many of these reforms were not implemented until eighty or ninety years later after the well-known Flexner Report of 1910 exposed many of the flaws in the system of medical education. Notably, Drake was the first to outline the stages of becoming a physician as being premedical, medical school, apprenticeship, first years in practice, and experienced physician.

Drake was a popular teacher. He knew his audience and was familiar with different methods of instruction that remain timeless. He was well organized, engaged learners with questions, used illustrative anecdotes, sustained interest with eloquent language, and was accessible to students. The selections in this section offer a sample of Drake's lessons as an educator and provide insight into his legacy as an eminent teacher.

4.1 BEGINNING AS A TEACHER

I am now going to astonish you so cling hold of every support within your reach—*I am a Professor!* Yes, incredible as it may appear to you and my other intimate friends, I am really and bona fide appointed a professor, and I repeat it on this side of the sheet, to save you the trouble turning back to see whether your eyes did not deceive you. I am, let me repeat, unquestionably a professor; but you must not suppose, by this, I am a great man. For a professorship to confer greatness, it must be a professorship in a great institution. But that does not happen to be the case in this instance. In Lexington, Kentucky, there has been for many years an incorporated seminary, styled Transylvania University. It has ample endowments, but very little celebrity. The trustees are, however, engaged in the erection of a large and elegant college edifice, and have established a faculty of medicine, as well as a faculty of the arts. The Professorship of *Materia Medica* and Botany is the one they have offered to me, and five days ago I signified my acceptance. I am not, however, about to move thither, but calculate to be suffered to spend my winters there, and the rest of the year in this place. You will, of course, feel alarmed for my professional interest here, but they are, I think, pretty well secured. My old master, Dr. Goforth, has returned to this place, and knowing his popularity, and that he would form a partnership with some person, I proposed such a connection with myself, on the first instance it commenced. He will attend to our united business in winter, and I shall, for two or three years, at least, be at liberty to pursue my studies without interruption. If the trustees should be displeased with my residing here, I will resign, as I have no wish to exchange Cincinnati for Lexington.

Excerpted from letter [circa 1817] cited in *The Life of Daniel Drake, by Edward Mansfield*. Cincinnati: Applegate & Co., 1855. 119–120.

READER REFLECTION

1. *Teaching is another way of adding value to those around you. Is this something that you would consider doing? Can you "teach" others even if not in a formal teaching position?*
2. *How does one get to be a good teacher?*

✂ 4.2 CHOOSING A GOOD TEACHER

I come now to the choice of preceptors. This is the point of more importance than most parents suppose. Many of them, indeed, seem to act on this important subject with but little discrimination. The circumspection with which they select masters, when about to apprentice their sons to mechanical occupations, is seldom manifested when a medical education is the object. They appear indeed to feel themselves incompetent to judge, in the latter case, and, generally, consult econo-my or convenience; although in so doing, they not infrequently determine for their sons, a far more imperfect and limited destiny than they intend.

1. It is not necessary that the preceptor should be a man of genius; but it is indispensable that he should *possess a sound and discriminating judgment*; otherwise he will be a blind guide. Of his qualifications in this respect, every parent with opportunities of personal intercourse may form a correct opinion. It is not requisite that he himself should be acquainted with the principles of the profession to judge of the talents and *common sense of its practitioners*: the most unlearned can distinguish between a clouded and an unclouded intellect.

2. A preceptor *should be learned, at least in his profession*. If the father wishes to make his son a skillful mechanic, he places him with the good workman—not a botch. How can a man direct the studies of a youth through the elements of several different sciences, if his acquaintance with them is imperfect and confused? As well might architecture be taught by one, who ignorantly combined in the same column, the parts and proportions which belong to all the different orders. To judge of the attainments of professional men is a more difficult task than to estimate their abilities; but although a father may not be able to do this by direct inquiries, he still has much in his power in this respect. *The previous opportunities of the individual whom he scrutinizes, taken in connection with his existing habits, will generally enable him to come to the correct conclusion.* If the former have been limited and the latter are idle, he may safely conclude, that the requisite attainments are wanting; and look elsewhere for the aid which is indispensable to rapid and logical prosecution of studies.

3. It is not sufficient that a private preceptor has talents and learning. *He must be devoted to his profession, jealous of its character, and ambitious of its honors.* With such feelings, he will awaken high aspirations in the bosom of the youth whose destiny is committed to his keeping, enamor him with the sciences whose rudiments he is to acquire, and animate him in the toil which their difficulties impose.

4. The preceptor *should be conscientious in the performance of his duties; that is, he should feel the responsibilities of his office, and studiously endeavor to discharge them.* It is easy to deceive the father in regard to the progress of a son, in the study of a profession with which the former is unacquainted, for all his partialities coincide with the flattering reports of the master, and cause them to be received with credulity. In this way many a tutor has repressed paternal anxiety, and screened, from paternal vigilance, his inattention and neglect; inspiring high hopes, at the

very moment when his own criminal derelictions of duty were sewing the seeds of their future destruction.

5. The primary preceptor should, if possible, be a man of business; *punctual to his pecuniary engagements, accurate in his accounts, and systematic in all his affairs.* He will thus be an example for the imitation of his pupils, on points in which too many students of medicine grow up with deplorable and enduring imperfections.

6. Finally, *sound morals and chastened habits* are not among the least of those qualifications, which an anxious father would require in the man, whose deportment and precepts are to exert so great an influence on the character of the son. It would be superfluous to numerate all vices, which ought to disqualify a physician for the private tuition of boys and young men; but there are a few which from their frequency and effect, deserve, on every suitable occasion, to be held up to the scorn of society. A want of attention to professional promises, with the consequent fabrication of excuses and apologies, is a failure which no preceptor can habitually display, with impunity to the morals of his pupil; and ought to be recorded regarded as a disqualification, with whatever genius and learning it might happen to be associated.

"Selection and Preparatory Education of Pupils." In *Practical Essays on Medical Education and the Medical Profession in the United States.* Cincinnati: Roff & Young, 1832. 21–23.

Reader Reflection

1. *What qualifications do you use to discriminate and assist with the choice of teachers/programs for yourself? How critical is this to success in your profession?*
2. *Think of the teachers and preceptors you have had. Did they live up to the principles Drake describes here? Who were your best teachers who had the most impact on you, and why?*

4.3 Specific Teaching Methods for Preceptors

I shall speak of the aid which the pupil should receive from his preceptor....

A well-directed superintendence [by a preceptor] will confer lasting benefits. The kind and manner of assistance must necessarily vary with the idiosyncrasies of both master and scholar; for that which facilitates the progress of one pupil, sometimes retards another, who requires a different regimen; and the methods which one preceptor follows with success, are often impractical for another, from being inconsistent with his temperament and habits. But in the midst of these diversities of character, to which an excessive importance ought not to be attached, we may perceive several methods which are applicable to every case, and I shall proceed to enumerate them.

1. The physician who proposes to become an instructor *shall provide the requisite books, engravings, preparations, and apparatus....*

2. He should *form a plan of elementary studies and require his pupil to follow it.* To this end he must designate every book that is to be read, and debar from them the perusal of any others. It is even necessary to mark portions which should be passed over, as being incomprehensible without ampler preparation, or as having been proven erroneous. All our systematic works abound in chapters of the latter kind, the study of which cannot be too strongly reprobated, as planting errors in the young mind which may never be eradicated.

3. He should *encourage his students to ask him questions and solicit his aid,* on the obscure and difficult parts of every author; that nothing may be passed through without being understood.

4. As a further means of effecting the same object, *he ought to examine every one on the book he has just finished*; and, thus, not only correct his errors, but animate him to close and accurate application.

5. At least once a week *he ought to assemble his pupils into a class, and subject them to systematic examinations on the studies they engaged.* When such examinations are ably conducted, they constitute the most interesting and valuable exercises in which students ever engage. By a series of well-directed questions he may guide them through the labyrinth of the most complicated subject; and enable them to analyze that which they would otherwise find impenetrable and hopeless. Their errors of principle and nomenclature will be corrected; and their confidence in the truth established; their scattered acquirements solidified into a system, its deficiencies made manifest, and the mode of supplying them indicated. Thus they will be led to contemplate and comprehend the relations which unite facts, that in badly educated minds remain insulated and in apparent variance. Above all, he can in this way and no other relieve the tedium of solitary reading; invest the study with charms that render it attractive; and inspire an emulation for relative excellence, that will seldom fail to work out positive distinction.

6. *He should require each pupil at least once a month to write a thesis* [i.e., reflection exercise]. This exercise should commence with his studies, and continue til it terminates in his inaugural dissertation. Its advantages are manifold, not the least of

which is the pleasure, which, in short time, it affords to every aspiring and inquisitive student. When studying anatomy, his thesis will of course be purely *descriptive*, kind of writing in which none can be proficient without practice. As he advances, they may assume a higher and more diversified character. Some of them will be simply *abridgments of chapters* written with diffuseness, of which, unfortunately there is no lack; others might be purely *analytical*; others *critical*, or in the *manner of reviews*; and a portion, mere *commentaries* on authors of a concise and *aphoristic* cast. In this way he will form habits of attention, and be led to study with profit, what he would have passed by with carelessness. In the latter periods of study, his essays may take on a still higher character. He may begin to unite facts into regular dissertations, according to the rules of a sound philosophical logic; investigating principles, and constructing the elements of the system which is to guide and govern his future efforts in the practice.

"Private Pupilage." In *Practical Essays on Medical Education and the Medical Profession in the United States.* Cincinnati: Roff & Young, 1832. 42–44.

Reader Reflection

1. *List the multiple approaches Drake suggests to engage the learner actively.*
2. *Consider the methods Drake proposes above—still useful and applicable? Were some of them included in your education? What was of greatest value to you? For learning on your own do you still use some of them? What methods have you found most personally useful?*

✴ 4.4 Using Experiments and Demonstrations to Teach

Experiments and demonstrations are, or should be, the great object, in every medical institution. Much that is taught in the lecture room might be as successfully studied elsewhere; but anatomy, chemistry, pharmacy, operative surgery, and obstetrics demand exhibitions to the eye, and no medical school is worthy of patronage, if deficient in the means of illustrating these important branches of the profession. Those, however, who endow and govern our institutions, should recollect, that the accumulation of the material of science cannot be made a substitute for skill in its use; and that a department loaded with apparatus will confer on students no substantial advantage, if the professor be deficient in talents and practical *tact*.

"Medical Colleges." In *Practical Essays on Medical Education and the Medical Profession in the United States.* Cincinnati: Roff & Young, 1832. 49.

Reader Reflection

1. As you prepare to learn something consider the best way to present or receive information to make it understandable and make it stick.

2. What complex ideas do you recall first getting exposed to through a demonstration or experiment that made it easier to understand those complex ideas?

4.5 Length of Terms and Limitations of Learning from Lectures

The late celebrated Professor [Caspar] Wistar admitted to me, in the year 1816, that the founders of the Philadelphia school had committed a great error in not establishing a session of six months, which would, doubtless, have been imitated by those who founded other institutions. The projector of the Medical College of Ohio [Drake] fixed its session at five months; which was, afterwards, unwisely reduced to four, although found to meet the approbation of the pupils. Were the different institutions of the United States to agree to extend their sessions to five or six months, they would do more to elevate the profession, than could be done by any other single act; and all who wish well to the dignity of the profession in the interests of humanity, should unite in affecting so desirable an object.

By extending the term, the existing evil of so many lectures each day would be obviated, and the student could find time to digest all that might be administered to him; as well as to compare what you should hear, with what you might see in the different text and standard works. Under existing circumstances, this is well known to be impracticable.

Four lectures a day are as many as can be appropriated to itself, by an ordinary mind, and the number should never exceed five. But few students can listen to six, with as much advantage as they would derive from two-thirds of that number. They become cloyed and oppressed; and long before the end of the fourth month, find themselves fatigued, impatient, and irritable, and prepare to depart. I have no doubt, that they would endure a session of six months, with fewer lectures, daily, in greater contentment, than they now bear our short sessions.

The daily succession of lectures, which requires attention of the student to pass, rapidly, from subject to subject, which have no natural relations to each other, is trying to the intellect of pupils, and necessarily detracts much from the value of our instruction.

"Medical Colleges." In *Practical Essays on Medical Education and the Medical Profession in the United States.* Cincinnati: Roff & Young, 1832. 47, 48.

Reader Reflection

1. *It seems obvious now—provide ample time for learners to reflect on what they are learning, space out lectures, have subjects that reinforce the content, and don't wear down the students. In your education was this done well, or could it have been improved?*

⊠ 4.6 Advice for Effective Lecturing

The faculty of awakening and sustaining the attention of an audience, is, in some degree, a gift of nature, and may be wanting, when other requisites are not. *An original or eccentric manner* is often the secret of success; *illustration* by means of anecdotes, skillfully introduced, produces the same effect; episodes may be so managed as to answer the purpose; *flights of fancy,* if well timed, will accomplish the end in view; while, in the absence of a talent for the whole of these, *unexpected and pertinent questions,* with familiar, conversational remarks, on the answers that maybe given, will resuscitate drooping energies of the class, enable them to hold out to the end....

A few questions on the matters which are to be immediately presented for examination will prepare the minds of the pupils for engaging in them, and can never fail to awaken the spirit of inquiry. During the lecture, interrogatories on the subject then before them are well calculated to arouse the attention of the students from [their] passive condition, and contribute greatly to relieve the tedium of their situation. But it is at the close that examinations are of the greatest value; as a recapitulation of the leading points will, in this manner, be indelibly impressed on the mind.

Medical professors should be men of learning, but the lecture room is not the most proper place to display the extent of their book researches. The citation of a great number of authorities is seldom profitable to students. They should expect from their teachers an account, clearly and methodically expressed, of the ascertained facts of the science; and, in general, the less this account is encumbered with quotations and references, the better will it be understood, and the deeper will be the impression. Great learning may excite the admiration of students; but their thirst for useful knowledge can only be satisfied by accurate analysis, and the school for arrangement of common and generally admitted facts....

Professors who speak *ex tempore*, have, in this respect, great advantage over those who read manuscripts, for the speaker must think, while the reader need not; and the class will generally follow their example. It has been objected to extemporary lectures, that they are apt to be repetitious, and deficient in method. Precision and arrangement, however, depend more on the mind of the teacher, than the circumstances under which his lectures are delivered.... Written lectures, moreover, are not easily altered, and once finished, are apt to be kept nearly in their original condition. Thus, what might have been as perfect, at first, as the state of the science permitted, is soon left behind, in the march of improvement; while the annual repetition of the same formula of words, diminishes the simplicity and force with which it is pronounced;

"And every year grows duller than the last."

"Medical Colleges." In *Practical Essays on Medical Education and the Medical Profession in the United States.* Cincinnati: Roff & Young, 1832. 50, 58–59.

Reader Reflection

1. *How many of your teachers often begin a lecture with questions or an anecdote and periodically pose more questions through the course of a lecture? How effective is this in keeping the learner's attention?*
2. *How can today's technology be used to engaged the student?*
3. *Assess your teachers: which ones teach to be admired? Any original or eccentric ones? And which teach for the student to learn?*

4.7 Have Learners Take Notes

Taking notes is an important employment of the lecture room, and one for which but few students are prepared. At the beginning of the course, most of them are zealous in this labor; but its difficulties, in many cases, speedily diminish this zeal, which is often succeeded by downright indifference....

In the last century, when the practice of publishing everything did not prevail, as in the present age, the necessity of making notes was much greater. There is a value, however, in this labor, distinct from the manuscript information at which it puts the student in possession. It in some degree secures and sustains his attention, and the extension and filling out of his notes, at his room, is a valuable exercise, leading to a kind of intellectual rumination, and favoring advancement in the important art of composition. Students, however, who can command their attention, and have retentive memories, would do well to write down but little, till they retire; when they should record such facts and principles as appear to be original or of great practical utility. In the perception of these, more, perhaps, than anything else, will the discriminating or instinctive sagacity of the pupil manifest itself. As students who write in the lecture room can only record a part of what is said, they should exercise a quick, and in loose phraseology, an intuitive judgment, as to what especially deserves to be recorded; otherwise in laboring upon the common-place, the new and valuable may entirely escape their attention.

"Medical Colleges." In *Practical Essays on Medical Education and the Medical Profession in the United States.* Cincinnati: Roff & Young, 53, 54.

READER REFLECTION

1. What is the value of taking notes manually in class? How does it reinforce learning?

4.8 INSPIRE THE LOVE OF LEARNING

The love of knowledge is not a desire, which we can press into our catalogue of principles to which we address our rewards and punishments; but goes very far to render them unnecessary; and may be placed high on the list of the preventive means of offences. It is then a great auxiliary to the teacher, but how is it inspired? As it is a duty to study, all the means enumerated as far as they can be used, may be employed, in turn to reward and punish him who is idle; but still the assigned lessons may be studied through *fear of punishment* and not *con amore*; and when the pupil leaves the institution, he may loathe the acquisition of further knowledge, even the more for having been punished into what he has acquired. Nevertheless, that which, to speak figuratively, has been whipped into the mind, is not without its use, as it has often happened, that he who at first studied only from fear, comes at length to study from love. Severity of punishment in these cases should, however, be the *ultima ratio praeceptoris* [tutor's last argument] and always connected with other means, calculated to awaken the dormant passion. The plan of this discourse does not carry us into the consideration of this subject, and I should be little qualified to illustrate it before a body of enlightened practical teachers; but I will throw out a few hints, although foreign in some degree to our immediate object. But are they in fact foreign? Will not the scholar study it if he derives pleasure from it? He undoubtedly will, and this pleasure will reward him, and incite him to renewed efforts. Let the teacher then secure him this pleasure, and it will generate the love of knowledge. But how, in many minds, can this be done? In some it *cannot* be done, for all the intellects are not equal; and some were never designed to comprehend the properties and relations of things. But omitting a reference to these, I would say, *First,*—that philosophical maxim—*pass from the known to the unknown,* should be observed, and that its violation has prevented many a scholar from acquiring a love of study; because he was put, carelessly or unskillfully, on such plans as rendered the acquisition of knowledge difficult or impossible. *Secondly*—Different minds are differently constituted, as to the balance among their faculties and tastes. One will have a strong talent for languages; another for the collecting and treasuring up historical facts; another for relations among natural bodies; and another for the idealities of imagination. But our plans of school classification do not recognize this important fact; and it must happen, that many are repulsed from study, and go through school or go from it, without acquiring a love of knowledge, simply by the influence of some branch, for which they had no capacity; who, if they had been tried separately, or in succession, on all the branches, might at length, have met with one, which was to their taste because adapted to their mental capability, and making progress in this, they would have passed by an easy transition to others, and finally acquired a love for the whole. *Third*—Something, I think may be done, by substituting the didactic conversation of the teacher, for the authors that are usually provided; as many things are rendered clear and attractive in colloquial intercourse, that seem obscure and incomprehensible in the formality of books. *Fourth*—It may be possible to arouse the dormant attention by showing the useful applications of knowledge of various kinds, in visits to works of art, where that knowledge manifests its utility and power. *Fifth*—Going into the great domain of nature, where every young heart palpitates more actively, and directing the attention of the pupil first, to curious and beautiful productions, as mere objects of sense; and then calling his awakened attention, to their structure, properties, and relations, as far as to excite his curiosity, and put his faculties of knowledge into action; and, *finally*, referring him for a full account to the books; which he may then be induced to read.

By means like these, I have seen a love of knowledge aroused in the minds of students of medicine; and, therefore, speak from some experience.

"Discipline: Discourse on the Philosophy of Family, School, and College Discipline." *Transactions of the Fourth Annual Meeting of the Western Literary Institute and College of Professional Teachers.* [Held in Cincinnati October 1834.] Cincinnati: Josiah Drake Publisher, 1835. 51, 52.

Reader Reflection

1. *Drake recommends that teachers start with what the student knows. Start with what is easiest for him/her. Show him/her how useful it is. Start with the senses. Think of a time when one of your teachers used each of these methods, and recall how it helped you acquire the love of learning.*
2. *What are the hindrances to developing the love of learning? How may we overcome them?*

4.9 Cultivate and Improve the Faculty of Observation

The student of medicine must cultivate the faculty of observation. No pursuit in life requires this faculty in equal perfection. The practice of medicine is the application of means to the attainment of definite ends, *those ends being ascertained by personal observation at the bedside of the sick.* Nearly all the senses are necessary to this observation and in a full practice (such as we intend you shall have) the time allotted to each patient is so short, that without habits of rapid and accurate observation, it will be impossible for you to come into possession of all the facts. *A faculty for quick and comprehensive observation is power.* It is time, for it bestows on its possessor both. He who possesses and exercises it, is efficient in the exact proportion, for the dispatch of business which it ensures, enables him daily to travel through the circle of professional duties, and have leisure for the cultivation of literature, auxiliary science, and the domestic and social relations. Thus he can accomplish more by the age of forty, than the unobserving and drowsy drone will have achieved at three score and ten. "Whatsoever the hand findeth to do, that do with all thy might" is an admirable maxim and founded on sound physiological principles. Rapid observation implies excited attention with acute sensibility, both of which are favorable to accuracy.

"The Formation of Professional Character" [1835]. In *Frontiersman of the Mind,* edited by Charles D. Aring. Cincinnati: History of the Health Sciences Library and Museum, University of Cincinnati, 1985.

READER REFLECTION

1. *How does a person develop his or her powers of observation? Discuss the sort of "power" it creates. Think of a time when one of your teachers showed you how to notice something that you were missing.*

2. *Do you agree that the ability to observe—which implies the ability to interpret and understand—is directly related to the physician's power in patient care?*

✖ 4.10 RECOGNIZE WHAT CAPACITIES STUDENTS NEED FOR A MEDICAL CAREER

Of the various occupations in society, scarcely one requires greater talent and knowledge, than the medical profession.... The ranks of the profession are in a great degree filled up with recruits, deficient either in abilities or acquirements— too often indeed in both—who thus doom it to a mediocrity, incompatible with both its nature and objects.

Few of those who are put to the study of medicine can be aware of the magnitude of the undertaking, or of the insufficiency of their capacity and preparation; for the obvious reason, that they are, in general, young and inexperienced...but it is not sufficient that individuals selected for the study of medicine should have good constitutions; they ought, equally, to be *endowed with vigorous and inquiring minds.* Without these, whatever may be the appearances of success, they must at least make incompetent physicians. It is especially and indispensably necessary, that they possess, in a high degree, *the faculties of observation and judgment*; without which, they can neither comprehend the principles of the science, nor apply them correctly in the treatment of diseases....

The student of medicine should not only be of *sound understanding,* but *imbued with ambition.* A mere love of knowledge is not to be relied upon, for the greatest lovers of knowledge are not infrequently deficient in executive talent, and go on acquiring without learning how to appropriate.... A thirst for fame is indeed a safer guarantee, and a taste for learning; as it generates those executive efforts, which are indispensable to the successful practice of the profession.

Further, the temperament of the youth should be that of *industry and perseverance*; without which he will bark at every difficulty, and require to be doted on through all stages of his pupilage.

Of all the causes which impede the progress of medicine in the United States, not one is more operative than this—ignorance on what is really necessary to make good physicians.

"Selection and Preparatory Education of Pupils." In *Practical Essays on Medical Education and the Medical Profession in the United States*. Cincinnati: Roff & Young, 1832. 5–8.

READER REFLECTION

1. *In your field what are the needed raw "human" materials to make a person successful? List those that Drake said is needed to become a good physician. How does that compare to what you believe is needed in your field?*

2. *How do you determine that a potential candidate for your field has the needed characteristics (character, capacities, abilities) to be successful?*

4.11 THE CARDINAL VIRTUES OF A STUDENT

A thorough course of preparatory learning is useful, in more ways than one. It establishes early habits of application; generates a love of knowledge; trains the faculties; and inspires that firmness of purpose, which prevents him to put his hand to the plow, from looking back. These are the cardinal virtues of the student; and they are in a great degree the effect of cultivation. We look instinctively at the grand and beautiful aspects of nature, but this is poetry, not philosophy. A poet delineates the surface, a philosopher decomposes the substance of things. One is born, the other called to his vocation. Education never made a great poet, nor nature a good philosopher. He is essentially the product of art. Toil is his destiny. He must sink a deep shaft and draw up his treasures from below. Therefore he should be strengthened by timely and active effort. He must be inured to labor, and acquire adroitness in his performance. Hence he should begin early, for then only can suitable habits be formed.

"Selection and Preparatory Education of Pupils." In *Practical Essays on Medical Education and the Medical Profession in the United States.* Cincinnati: Roff & Young, 1832. 17.

READER REFLECTION

1. *What did you take from your preparatory learning that was critical to your subsequent development?*
2. *Consider Drake's "cardinal virtues" of a student and their relevance today.*

⊠ 4.12 APPRECIATE THE VALUE OF LATIN AND GREEK LANGUAGES AND KNOWLEDGE OF THE ANCIENT TEXTS

A physician who is ignorant of the Latin and Greek languages, whatever may be his genius and professional skill, must, to the eye of sound scholarship, appear defective and uncultivated. For more than 2000 years, these languages, especially the former, were the vehicles of all medical knowledge, except a little contributed by the Arabians; and, till within a century, our professional ancestors wrote, and prescribed, and thought, and lectured, in Latin. It was, indeed, to the profession a universal language; affording the means of an easy and accurate correspondence, among all the schools and physicians of Europe. Even down to the present time, the lectures in most of the Italian and German Universities were delivered in Latin; while the examination of candidates, in many others, is conducted in the same language. Thus it has had the most protracted and intimate companionship with medicine; to the nomenclature of which it has freely lent its opulent vocabulary. Many of its words, no doubt, as well as those drawn from the dialects of Greece, are intended to convey, in their new situation, ideas materially different from their vernacular import; but in attempting to understand even these, the student is greatly assisted by acquaintance with their primitive significations. With this knowledge of our dependence on the languages and literature of the ancients, to deny that the study of them must be beneficial, is scarcely less absurd, then to affirm, on the other hand, that every classical scholar is of necessity of physician.

"Selection and Preparatory Education of Pupils." In *Practical Essays on Medical Education and the Medical Profession in the United States.* Cincinnati: Roff & Young, 1832. 16.

Reader Reflection

1. *Every profession has a history and has specific foundational knowledge on which it rests. What are the key historical developments of your profession?*
2. *How does knowing the historical basis of your profession benefit you?*

⊠ 4.13 Stages to Professional Excellence

In the preceding essay, on the preparatory education of students, I have endeavored to show, that its errors and imperfections are permanently stamped on our literary character. If this be the fact, we can scarcely doubt, that a defective elementary education, in medicine, must greatly retard our advancement to professional excellence; and whatever does this, demands the gravest attention.

The ordinary time of private instruction is so short, as to require that it should be well employed. If the rudiments of the profession are then acquired, they are seldom properly understood. It is not easy, afterwards, to supply the omissions, or correct the errors of that period. I have never known it done. Every stage of life has its peculiar taste and appropriate studies. In youth we acquire elementary truths. In manhood we arrange them into general principles. In the meridian of life, we apply them to the production of practical results. Such is the law of nature; and was it inscribed on the doors of every medical library, they would not so often be opened to no beneficial effect.

"Selection and Preparatory Education of Pupils." In *Practical Essays on Medical Education and the Medical Profession in the United States.* Cincinnati: Roff & Young. 1832. 17.

Reader Reflection

1. *There are clear stages professionals progress through to get to excellence. Consider the stages for your discipline and what "studies" are necessary in each stage that is needed to advance to the next.*

⊠ 4.14 Train for Frequent Interruptions

The situations and circumstances in which a pupil should prosecute his studies, deserve to be considered. In the country and all the small towns of the United

States, the fashion is for the student to reside and study in the shop or office of his preceptor, and often to become a member of his family. The latter has its advantages, as contributing to preserve him from dissipation; but his time is too often wasted in labors foreign to his studies; he is apt to be introduced more frequently into company, than is compatible with his interests as a student. Of the office, as a place for study, "much might be said on both sides." It is the resort of many persons for those who call for medical assistance, and the student is subjected to perpetual, if not protracted interruptions. In this way he loses many precious hours, which could never be reclaimed. At first, the effect of these interruptions is so distracting, as materially to impede his progress; but their influences diminishes with the repetition, until at last he comes to form habits that are not without their value in after life. To understand this, we need only recollect, *that the practice of his profession will subject him to incessant interruptions of a similar kind*; if he has not early acquired the art of reading in the midst of them, he will not read at all. From the want of this habit, many physicians pass their lives incapable, as they conceive, from the vexations of business, of reading as many volumes as they should study every year.

"Selection and Preparatory Education of Pupils." In *Practical Essays on Medical Education and the Medical Profession in the United States*. Cincinnati: Roff & Young, 1832. 25.

READER REFLECTION

1. *In some career fields, for example, medicine, interruptions are part of the workflow. How does a person train to give full attention to what is at hand and not get easily distracted?*

✖ 4.15 MANAGE THE DAY

The portion of each day, which pupils in medicine may devote to their studies, consistently with good health in the future welfare of their constitutions, must necessarily vary in different persons; but a safe average would be 1/2, or 12 hours. This would give seven for sleep—and few young persons can do with less—two for meals, and three for exercise, labor, and society. The last of these divisions is abridged by some and lengthened by others; but in general is profitless to all. With most pupils, the hours of relaxation from study are hours of idleness, pleasure, and gossip: too often of downright listlessness or ruinous dissipation. But whether whiled or rioted away, they bring no renovation either of mind or body. To answer the end for which they are set apart, they must be spent in active exertion in the open air; which will not only prepare the mind for new laborers, but ward off dyspepsia, palpitations, hypochondraism, and red eyes; and prevent that debility of frame, so falsely regarded as the necessary effect of hard study, when it results from the want of a sufficient amount of hard labor.

"Private Pupilage." In *Practical Essays on Medical Education and the Medical Profession in the United States*. Cincinnati: Roff & Young, 1832. 26, 27.

Reader Reflection

1. *Have you discovered a daily schedule that leads to optimal effectiveness? What is it?*

4.16 Take Care of Yourself during Your Student Days

Students when in attendance on lectures, should look carefully to the preservation of their health. The new causes which may impair it, are, first, a more inactive and sedentary life; secondly, a fuller and more stimulating diet, than most of them have been accustomed to at home; thirdly, a change in hours of eating, especially, breakfast and dinner, both of them being too late—the former for an obvious reason, the latter, because, the appetite becomes importunate, and leads to gastric repletion; fourthly, in many cases abridgment of the hours of sleep; fifthly, intense and perplexing application of mind; sixthly, crowded and badly ventilated lodging rooms; finally, dissipated pleasures, into which they are too often seduced by all the allurements of the great cities, the common and most proper sites for medical institutions. From the operation of these, and other causes, the health of medical students, during the session, is exceedingly apt to become impaired. The maladies to which they are most liable are constipation, hepatic torpor and engorgement, dyspepsia, headache, chronic ophthalmia, palpitation of the heart, hypochondriasm, ennui [listlessness], jactatition [restless tossing], fidgets, and other forms of nervous irritation. With any of these maladies upon him, the student will make sorry progress; most of them, however, might be prevented, by temperance, exercise in the open air, and general regularity of life and conduct.

"Medical Colleges." In *Practical Essays on Medical Education and the Medical Profession in the United States*. Cincinnati: Roff & Young, 1832. 57–58.

READER REFLECTION

1. *Which factors causing poor health in students listed here still apply?*
2. *What is Drake's advice for preserving your health during your student days?*

✶ 4.17 SET ASIDE TIME TO DEVELOP YOUR CHARACTER

Is it necessary that the student of medicine should prosecute his studies on Sunday? And answering this question, I shall of course speak not as a divine, but a physician and teacher. I would say, then, that it is not, but the reverse. As a general rule, his progress will be greater, if he suspend, and not continue his studies to the Sabbath. The mind, not less than the body, requires not mere moments of relaxation but hours of actual repose, at least from the particular labors in which it is engaged. Moreover, the student comes into his medical pupilage with established habits in this respect, which cannot be violated with advantage. Finally, the moral and devotional feelings require cultivation, and this can best be done by the occurrence, at stated times, of a day for that special object. On the whole, therefore, I regard those preceptors, who encourage their pupils in the prosecution of medical studies on the Sabbath, as committing an error in their plan of professional education.

"Private Pupilage." In *Practical Essays on Medical Education and the Medical Profession in the United States.* Cincinnati: Roff & Young, 1832. 27.

READER REFLECTION

1. *Consider the benefits of taking a weekly break from your work. How do you spend your time to reenergize?*
2. *A person's character contributes significantly to success. What does "character" mean to you? Do you spend time reflecting on your character and the direction it is heading? How does a person become an individual of great character?*

✶ 4.18 ACQUIRE THE HABIT OF MANAGING YOUR MONEY AND LIFESTYLE WELL

Few things exert a greater influence on our prosperity than a systematic attention to pecuniary accounts, and the observance of a judicious economy in our expenditures; all of which must be practiced in youth, to become matters of habit and manhood. When a father sends his son from home to study the profession, he should decide upon the style of living (always simple and unostentatious) in which the young man is to pass in his apprenticeship; and furnishing him, from time to time, with the necessary means, should require of him to render at stated periods an account of their appropriation. This would compel him not only to limit his expenditures to his resources, but give him, at an early period, a habit of recording his disbursements and keeping his accounts, that would be a great advantage in all after years. I have known many physicians, who were neither accurate accountants nor good economists, clearly because they have grown up in the habitual neglect of the duties which I have indicated.

"Private Pupilage." In *Practical Essays on Medical Education and the Medical Profession in the United States*. Cincinnati: Roff & Young, 1832. 20.

Reader Reflection

1. *Consider your habits of managing your money. How did you acquire these habits? Is managing your money a source of worry for you?*
2. *What new habits could you acquire to minimize the worry about money?*

4.19 Get a Liberal Arts Education with a Daily Habit

Other studies than medicine should occupy a portion of the students' time. In the preceding essay, I have said that a majority of our students of medicine, particularly those of the West, enter upon their pupilage with the most incompetent education. For all such there is no alternative, but to cultivate the elements of literature and science during their medical pupilage, or to remain superficial scholars throughout their lives. I regret to say that the majority choose the latter. But are those who have enjoyed the advantages of a collegiate education exempted from the necessity which rests upon their less favored brethren? It is obvious that they have not. Few minds are so retentive as to keep what they have acquired at school, if they do not add to it, by a subsequent cultivation of the same branches. *To secure this important object, it is absolutely necessary, that the student should devote to it a steady portion of every day—for example in the morning or evening*; and suffer no controllable circumstances to interfere with his plan. A small part of his time thus occupied, well in the course of four or five years make him a passable scholar, should his learning have even been at the minimum; but when he has the happiness to engage in professional studies with the attainment of a bachelor, he may by the course here recommended, so far extend his literary requirements, as to enter on the theater of life with an enviable character for sound erudition.

"Private Pupilage." In *Practical Essays on Medical Education and the Medical Profession in the United States.* Cincinnati: Roff & Young, 1832. 28–29.

Reader Reflection

1. *Consider how a goal of becoming a scholar may contribute to creating your legacy.*
2. *Is becoming a scholar important in your career development? What is required to become a "passable scholar"?*

4.20 Recognize How Other Fields of Learning Can Inform and Assist Your Work

The student of medicine should devote a portion of his time to the following principal branches of literature and science:

First, English grammar and the art of composition; without an attention to it, after the commencement of his medical studies, no young man need hope to become even a tolerable writer.

Secondly, physical geography, embracing leading facts in meteorology, which constitutes a foundation for the study of physical condition and diseases of man, and the various countries and climates of the earth; a comprehensive view which should be taken by every physician.

Thirdly, the outline of history; that he may be able to trace the progress of the profession through the different nations which have transmitted it to his own; and come to understand the influence of moral causes on the physical system, whose aberrations he is to rectify.

Fourthly, the elements of mathematics and natural philosophy; not merely for the purpose of invigorating his reasoning powers, but because the latter has many points of illustrative association with medicine.

Fifthly, the French language; since the subjects of morbid anatomy, physiology pathology, have been recently cultivated with extraordinary success by the French physicians; but a small part of whose voluminous and classical writings are translated into our vernacular tongue. To avail himself of this source of improvement, it is not necessary that the students should conquer the difficulties of the French pronunciation. A few elementary books, with or without a teacher, are all that are requisite to open to him the rich treasures of medical knowledge, which that enterprising people have accumulated.

Sixthly, Latin and Greek languages. Of all the branches of literature which have been named, it is, perhaps, most necessary, for those who would retain or establish the character of good scholars, to continue the study of these languages, through the period of their medical pupilage.

"Selection and Preparatory Education of Pupils." In *Practical Essays on Medical Education and the Medical Profession in the United States.* Cincinnati: Roff & Young, 1832.

READER REFLECTION

1. *Any field has a core body of knowledge, but Drake reminds us that other fields of study can contribute to a person's future effectiveness and success. Consider your own career field: What fields of study relate to it in some way or could be of practical use to your career?*

🞛 4.21 PRINCIPLES FOR LEARNING AND BUILDING A FOUNDATION FOR YOUR PROFESSION

Consider the plan on which the pupil should be conducted through his professional studies. "Method," says Linnaeus, "is the soul of science," an apothegm to which most private preceptors in this country seem to be strangers.... In medicine, as in the other sciences, that method is best, which requires the student to take nothing on trust—to anticipate [assume] no principal or leading fact....

...[H]e ought to begin with chemistry; it is not necessary, however, that he should go extensively or minutely into the practical details of the science, for the object is merely to prepare him for a proper understanding of the chemical terms, with which he will meet in the study of physiology.

Relinquishing chemistry he should engage in special anatomy, which may be studied in the following order: one—the bones, two—the muscles, three—the viscera, four—the blood and absorbent vessels, five—the brain and nerves. He is now prepared for general anatomy, and should make himself familiar to anatomical relations and dependence of the various organs.

He will thus qualify himself for the study of physiology, and the foundations of which are anatomy and chemistry; and his progress, in that important branch of the profession, will, *ceteris paribus* [holding other things constant], be in proportion to the accuracy of his anatomical and chemical knowledge.... The close of his physiological course, will embrace the philosophy of mind; a branch of science, if science it can as yet be called, whose dignity, and undeniable connection with the study of mental alienation, may compensate for the obscurity of its data and the uncertainty of its deductions.

From Physiology he may either recur to the studies of which chemistry is the basis, or, according to his taste or the judgment of his teacher, proceed by natural transition to acquire an outline of Pathology. The latter is perhaps, on the whole, the better course; for when the mind of a pupil is deeply interested in the contemplation of the healthy functions, it passes with facility to the study of their disordered states; and thus, with little difficulty, comes to comprehend the general principles of pathology. But he should, on no account, be permitted to stray beyond the rudiments of the science of diseased actions. And here I will take occasion to remark, that I know of no distinct treatise on the elements of pathology which is adapted to this stage of a pupil's studies.

"Private Pupilage." In *Practical Essays on Medical Education and the Medical Profession in the United States.* Cincinnati: Roff & Young, 1832. 30–32.

READER REFLECTION

1. *There is a sequence that aids in the acquisition of a growing base of knowledge. For your field what is the sequence of foundational knowledge?*
2. *Method brings order to chaos and is fundamental to learning. What is your method for learning? How do you learn best—where knowledge is retained, and you are equipped to use it?*

4.22 CONSIDER THE BEST SETTING FOR LEARNING SPECIFIC TYPES OF KNOWLEDGE

Every student...should spend a part of his pupilage among the officinal substances [herbs or drugs] that are the agents with which future objects are to be accomplished. He should learn their sensible qualities by observation, and become familiar with all the compounds and pharmaceutical processes of the shop. But to acquire this knowledge, it is only necessary that he should be in the office, or in the shop of an apothecary, while prosecuting the study of chemistry and pharmacy. When engaged in anatomy, physiology, pathology, and botany, the dissecting room, his chamber, and the field, are his appropriate situations. After having, however, acquired competent knowledge of those branches, with the principles of surgery in the classification of diseases, he may and should return to the scenes of practical medicine; he is then prepared to comprehend the nature of what he sees, and to a certain extent, can engage understandingly in the duties of the profession.

"Private Pupilage." In *Practical Essays on Medical Education and the Medical Profession in the United States.* Cincinnati: Roff & Young, 1832. 26.

Reader Reflection

1. *As a student or teacher how do you create or establish a favorable context/environment, e.g., reinforcing experiences, for learning?*
2. *Consider which environment/setting is needed to best learn knowledge, skills, and/or adopt new attitudes?*

4.23 Training for a Special Area: Learning Surgery

Should the student intend to make operative surgery his principal object he may... [pay] special attention on the following subjects:

1. *Anatomy of the parts* which are the seats of the greater operations of the art. With these parts, particularly such of them as cannot be cut into without danger, he should be perfectly familiar: not merely able to enumerate the muscles, and fascia, the nerves, and blood vessels of which they are composed, but to conceive accurately of the relative situation of those anatomical elements. He should, moreover, *learn to know each part, not only by the eye, but by the finger*; as it will frequently happen, in deep and bloody operations, that the sense of touch is the only one he can employ.

2. He should *practice the various operations on the dead subject*; for by practice only, can he become adroit, or acquire that confidence which gives self possession in moments of difficulty and doubt. In this stage of his practical studies, he will often find it advantageous to supply the deficiency of human subjects, by a resort to dead

animals; in the selection of which he will be materially aided by some acquaintance with zoology.

3. He should *practice on the living or the dead subject, the application of the various kinds of bandages and apparatus of surgery.* For the neat and efficient discharge of this duty, more experience is necessary, than many persons suppose until they come to the trial in cases of real injury, when it is too late to prepare themselves.

"Private Pupilage." In *Practical Essays on Medical Education and the Medical Profession in the United States.* Cincinnati: Roff & Young, 1832. 40.

READER REFLECTION

In 1832 there were no formal surgical training programs in the United States. What Drake recommended here did not formally occur until sixty years later with Dr. William Halsted at the Johns Hopkins Hospital.

1. *What are the fundamentals you need to practice to reach a level of mastery in your field?*
2. *What does Drake mean when he says, "learn to know each [body] part, not only by the eye, but by the finger"?*
3. *What innovations would you bring to teaching in your field?*

✖ 4.24 DIAGNOSIS IS LEARNED AT THE BEDSIDE

It is in hospitals, that the lectures on practical or clinical medicine must be delivered. To hear these and witness the cases to which they relate, would be an object with every student who might attend the Medical College.

An Inaugural Discourse on Medical Education. [Delivered at the opening of the Medical College of Ohio, Cincinnati, Ohio, November 11.] Cincinnati: Looker, Palmer, and Reynolds, 1820.

The subject of hospital practice must not be passed over in silence. That it might be made a source of great improvement to students, no one can deny; that it is such, no one, I believe, will venture to assert. For a few weeks after the commencement of the course of lectures, students are zealous in their attendance at the hospital, on prescribing days; but each one soon discovers, that in the throng, his opportunities for accurate personal observations on the condition of the sick are too few and momentary to render his attendance in the wards of any substantial benefit; and his visits, thenceforward, become occasional and still more unproductive, because made under a feeling of discouragement. To derive benefit from hospital practice, students, who have the means, should attend upon it through the vacation, when the number is smaller, and opportunities for personal observation are, consequently, much greater.

"Medical Colleges." In *Practical Essays on Medical Education and the Medical Profession in the United States.* Cincinnati: Roff & Young, 1832. 49.

It is the duty of the preceptor, when his pupil is prepared for clinical observation, to select for him such cases as will be profitable. The diagnosis of diseases presents many difficulties, and can be successfully studied only at the bedside. To introduce a student indiscriminately to all cases is more likely to confuse than enlighten his mind. He should first study those which present a well-defined character, and proceed gradually to the more obscure and complicated. But the most judicious selection of cases will impart but little instruction, unless they are made the subject of conversation and comment by the preceptor. In these clinical lectures, the benefit which he confers upon his disciple, if not greater, will be more deeply felt, then in any other period of their connection. The utility of what has been teaching will now be made apparent; and the enduring relation finally dissolved, with feelings of gratitude in one, and self-approving consciousness in the other.

"Private Pupilage." In *Practical Essays on Medical Education in the Medical Profession in the United States.* Cincinnati: Roff & Young, 1832. 44.

READER REFLECTION

1. *Teaching in the hospital was rare in the United States in 1820 and also 1832. At that time there were no rotations and no responsibility for the student. Drake recognized that learning clinical medicine occurs at the patient's bedside nearly sixty years before William Osler introduced this at the Johns Hopkins Hospital. Why do you think institutions struggle with making changes in how learners are educated?*
2. *Drake offers an important principle for teachers—begin with manageable information and skills before moving learners to more complex knowledge and tasks. Consider a complex task you are learning and begin to break it down into achievable steps.*

⊠ 4.25 Know the Leading Edge of Learning

Whatever, then, may be the ultimate aims of different pupils, their pathological studies should be the same. They must seek to acquire distinct and vivid conceptions of the morbid states which are supposed to be indicated by the terms congestion, irritation, inflammation, fever, nervous irritation, morbid sensibility, sympathy, spasm, morbid secretion, metastases, vicarious action, collapse, torpor, debility, exhaustion, proximate cause, organic lesion, *vis medicatrix* [the body's natural ability to heal itself], obstruction, local determination, malignity, and many others of subordinate moment, which constitute the elements of pathology, whether clinical or surgical. When they have grappled for sufficient time with the difficulties which every attempt to learn the true import of these common, but equivocal words unavoidably imposes, they may proceed to consider the varieties of inflammation, fever, spasm, and the other morbid states, which will bring them to Nosology, or the classification of diseases; when for the first time, they will perceive the paths by which those who intend to limit themselves to clinical medicine, and those who propose to cultivate operative surgery, are to diverge from each other. Having looked into the systems of Nosology, with sufficient care to perceive both their importance and their imperfections, the coadjutors [those who work together with another] may betake themselves in some degree to separate studies: the student of physic to functional, the student of surgery to organic derangements. The latter are, however, in all cases—mechanical injuries excepted—the offspring, as in turn they become the occasion, of the former; and hence they must both be studied by each class of pupils, though not in an equal degree. In his nosological inquiries, the student becomes acquainted with what the naturalist call central characters; but, arriving at the investigation of particular maladies, either medical or surgical, he will of course extend and correct his knowledge of symptomatology; endeavoring by the upmost of his understanding to connect each symptom with a morbid state of which it is the sign. In doing this he will be led to enlarge his knowledge of Morbid Anatomy, the first ideas of which might have been received while engaged on general pathology.

In this stage of his progress, he is qualified to investigate the causes of disease, the subject so enveloped in obscurity that many students give it but a passing attention. Aetiology is, however, a branch of medical science of sufficient importance to justify, I should rather say, demand an attentive investigation: and the very difficulties with which it is beset, should stimulate a pupil to its deep and protracted examination. Scarcely any portion of his studies will bring into requisition all his knowledge of nature and art, like that of which I am speaking. Of the origin, combination and mode of action of the *causis morborum* [causes of disease], much remains undeveloped; partly from the intrinsic difficulty of the subject, still more from the loose and limited manner in which it has been generally studied. With these convictions, I would indicate it to students of medicine, as a department of the profession in which they may labor with a well-founded hope of doing good to society and credit to themselves.

Finally, he arrives, by regular transition, at the practice of the profession—its therapeutics and operations. He studies the indications of cure, and labors to establish in his mind, correct associations between symptoms and remedies—an association not arbitrary and empirical, but founded on ample and accurate knowledge of the functions of the living body, in their regular and irregular conditions; and of the influence of external agents in the production and cure of diseases.

"Private Pupilage." In *Practical Essays on Medical Education and the Medical Profession in the United States.* Cincinnati: Roff & Young, 1832. 36, 37.

READER REFLECTION

1. *Every field has its own unique vocabulary. Here Drake maps out the major headings related to a new field of pathology. In 1832 there were no textbooks in pathology and it was not until 1840 when Drake's colleague Samuel Gross wrote the first US textbook on pathology. Do you have a map or "big picture" of your field? What approach(es) could you take to grow your field's technical vocabulary?*

✷ 4.26 HOW TO LEARN IN PRACTICE

Every part of a course of medical studies abounds in difficulties, and calls for intense and sustained application; but no stage is so trying to the powers of the student, as to that which may be called the Therapeutic [i.e., treatment]. Hitherto he has occupied himself, successively, upon distinct sciences, which he perceived to abound in connections favorable to that union into a system of professional knowledge; and that union, in reference to his own mind, he is now to effect. He is faithfully represented by the commander, who having embodied and equipped a variety of separate military corps, has at length to consolidate them into an army and direct its active operations.

It is difficult to furnish a student with rules for the organization of his various attainments into a practical system, and much must necessarily be left to his own genius and judgment. A few hints, however, may not be without their utility.

1. *If he now finds deficiencies* in any of his preliminary acquirements, he should apply them, without delay, by recurrence to the branches in which they are discovered to exist.

2. In ascertaining general principles, he should carefully *note those which are of a doubtful character*, and rest upon them as few rules of practice as possible.

3. His *practical maxims, in all cases, should be logical deductions* from his principles.

4. If they do not conform to those of the great and original writers of the profession, he should doubt their correctness, and act upon them cautiously; but *not reject them without a trial*.

5. He should recollect that the same diseases, in different countries, frequently require variation in their treatment, that he *must not implicitly adopt the rules of practice that have been found successful elsewhere*.

6. When he meets, in practical works, with different modes of treatment for the same disease, he *should not suppose that one can only be correct*, and the others necessarily erroneous, for diseases may be cured by various methods. Becoming an eclectic, in these cases, he must carefully examine the whole, and *test their merits by the great principles of pathology and therapeutics, which compose his own system*. When he attempts to select from among them, he should avoid uniting rules or recipes that are incompatible, and would therefore countervail or neutralize each other.

7. In his *practical readings*, he should always prefer original works to compilations, and monographs to systems.

8. He must be on his *guard against the delusion of a fancied simplicity* in the system with he constructs. Every complex machine is liable to a variety of irregular movements, which can only be reduced to order by a corresponding diversity of means. But of all machines the human body is the most complicated, exhibits the greatest number of disordered actions, all different from each other, and requires the greatest variety of remedial applications.

9. When he arrives at this stage in his studies he should know longer stand aloof from the practical duties of the profession; but *avail himself of frequent opportunities to make an application of his knowledge*. This is the end for which he has studied, and his final success will be proportionate to the facility and effect with which he can make such application. Skill in practice does not arise, however, from the number of cases he may see or treat, *so much as the manner in which he contemplates them*. Each one should

be a study, and all things related to it, should be connected with the principles to guide him, and which, in turn, they may serve to illustrate or overthrow.

"Private Pupilage." In *Practical Essays on Medical Education and the Medical Profession in the United States.* Cincinnati: Roff & Young, 1832. 38–40.

READER REFLECTION

1. *Drake recognized that each physician must acquire a comprehensive picture of how the extensive areas of medical knowledge and skills fit together in the person of the physician so that they can be applied in the care of the patient. How does a person build that comprehensive picture for him/herself? How are Drake's rules for learning in practice helpful to you?*

2. *Do other careers or fields have the same issue?—building the big picture? Is this one of the steps to mastery?*

❖ 4.27 STAGES OF MASTERY: MANY FIELDS HAVE COMPLEX PROBLEMS TO SOLVE

I shall attempt to illustrate and enforce what has been said on the magnitude and difficulties of the [medical] profession, by a short history of the employments and responsibilities of a medical man in this country, *where the various branches* [of learning] *are united in the same person.*

Let us suppose him to be called upon as an operator in *surgery*. He must be able to determine whether the age, health, and condition of his patient will admit of the operation; he should have an accurate knowledge of the structure of the parts through which his incisions are to be made, and be acquainted with the variety of instruments that have been employed, so as to select those which are best adapted to the particular case; he should know the history of the operation, and be qualified to choose from among the various modes that have been proposed for performing it, the easiest and most successful. Should any anomaly of structure lead to the injury of parts which cannot be cut without danger, it becomes his duty, suddenly, to decide upon and employ the means which are necessary to the preservation of life; and this he must do in the midst of general consternation, when deafened with the cries, and drenched in the gushing blood, of his patient—circumstances which require an accurate knowledge of the surrounding parts and quick powers of invention, not less than a firm and unshaken hand. Finally, the operation being over, and every accidental difficulty removed, he must determine on the means which should be employed to avert the dangerous symptoms that may result from an extensive mechanical injury, and secure the final recovery of his patient.

Suppose at another time he is called to *treat a malignant fever*. He has then to encounter a case of general disease; all parts of the complicated machine have been invaded; every organ has its functions deranged; and every fiber vibrates with a morbid action. Prompt and energetic efforts must be made, but these according to the causes and character of the disease may be of opposite kinds. What an important and difficult decision is then devolved upon him. The remote causes of malignant fevers must be considered; but these are uncertain and obscure, and the study of them involves a knowledge of secret changes in the earth and the atmosphere, that can neither be detected nor understood by those who are ignorant of the science of Chemistry. The symptoms of the disease are its language; but they speak intelligibly to him only, who has, by a long and arduous course of study and observation, established in his mind the relations which exist between external appearances and internal changes of action and structure; and who, from his previous knowledge of the laws of the human body in health, can determine, from visible signs, how far, and in what manner they have been violated in disease. Having thus, by the lights of Anatomy, Physiology, Chemistry, and Pathology, discovered the causes and character of the fever, it remains for him to decide upon its treatment. To fix upon the best, he should previously have acquired an accurate knowledge of the various plans of cure, which have been proposed in different ages and nations. He should be able to choose the most appropriate of these, and to modify it for the particular case under consideration. This will open to him a new duty, the selection, preparation, and administration of medicines: the able performance of which requires a knowledge of the effects of the various remedies on the body, both in health and disease; in other words, an acquaintance with Materia Medica, and certain parts, at least, of its subordinate and contributing sciences—Pharmacy, Botany, Mineralogy, and Zoology.

Again, suppose he is consulted for a *chronic malady of some internal organ*, on which the powers of medicine have been exhausted ineffectually, and the important question of a change of climate and country is proposed. How can he determine in what region his patient may find a condition of soil, water, and climate favorable to recovery, without a knowledge of Geology, Geography, and Meteorology?

Finally, he may be called to a *maniac*, and in the sad combination of mental and bodily disease, be presented with a case that requires him to possess a knowledge of the laws which regulate the mysterious influences of the mind and body upon each other. He will then perceive the necessity of an acquaintance with Metaphysics; for without it he must be utterly incapable of "administering to a mind diseased."

It would be easy to extend this exposition of the duties of a physician; but enough has been said, I trust, to prove, that no other profession requires in its practitioners so profound a knowledge of very different sciences,—such a versatility of mental effort, such an association of ideas apparently the most distant from each other,—such a power of calling up dormant facts,—such nice discrimination in the selection of precedents,—so collected a mind in moments of unexpected difficulty,—and so ready a resort to expedients, when established means are unattainable, or not adapted to the end in view.

An Inaugural Discourse on Medical Education. [Delivered at the opening of the Medical College of Ohio, Cincinnati, Ohio, November 11.] Cincinnati: Looker, Palmer, and Reynolds, 1820.

READER REFLECTION

1. *What are the complex or perplexing problems in your field? What knowledge is needed to solve those problems—some of which may not be in your original field of study?*
2. *Consider how addressing or solving them can contribute to your legacy.*
3. *What knowledge gaps have surfaced for you on the job?*

✖ 4.28 STAGES OF MASTERY: THE PHYSICIAN AS SCIENTIST, PHILOSOPHER, SCHOLAR, AND ARTIST

Literature and science are not the same; but a physician should acquire both, and the cultivation of the former ought to precede that of the latter. It is, however, a mortifying fact, that in the United States, and especially west of the mountains, the young men designed for the medical profession are in general destitute of this preparation in literature, so essential to their future acquisitions in science. Commencing the latter while ignorant of the former, their progress is comparatively slow and imperfect; and they learn, when too late, that a magnificent edifice cannot be erected on a narrow and badly constructed foundation. No young man should commence the study of medical science till he is at least sixteen years of age; and unless the preceding time have been devoted to the acquisition of language and the rudiments of general knowledge, he will neither possess that learning, nor those disciplined habits of application, that are essential to a successful prosecution of medical studies. While the standard of literary and professional excellence necessarily participated in the general imperfection which attended the institutions of our new country, this want of preparation in those who undertook the study of medicine was less striking, and had to be excused, from, being unavoidable. The opportunities for prosecuting a better course of preliminary studies have been created, even in the western states, and no young man should hereafter be encouraged to become a student of medicine, who has not prepared himself in a manner corresponding with the vast extent and inherent dignity of that science. This preparation should not consist merely in a detached knowledge of his own language. He should ascend to its ancient sources, and drink deeply at its pure and original fountains. If the principles of medical science, which are now taught, be not the same, that prevailed in Greece and Rome, they are partly expressed in the language of those learned and polished nations; and to be thoroughly understood, the words in which they are conveyed must themselves be made an object of study. So deeply impressed are the Faculty of this institution with the neglect of these studies, and the importance of them to the advancement and elevation of the profession, that they have offered an annual prize medal for the best inaugural thesis in the Latin language; and hope by this measure to excite among the students of the west an emulation for excellence in classical literature.

I have now made a rapid enumeration of the various branches of literature and science, which a physician should regard as indispensable, or important, objects of cultivation. *By proper attention to these, the student may become a philosopher and scholar; but something more will be necessary to make him a successful practitioner of medicine.* He must not only comprehend the principles of the profession; but, by acute and patient observation at the bedside of the sick, learn how to apply them in the cure of diseases. *He has to make himself an artist*; but his skill must consist in the practical application of the precepts and maxims of science. Clinical medicine, is an unceasing employment of means for the accomplishment of specific or definite objects: Considered in relation to our knowledge of those means, the [medical] profession is a science—*in relation to the application of them, it is an art.* He who acquires the former only, is learned; he who relies on the latter alone, is ignorant, empirical and criminal; he who compasses both, reaches the highest attainable perfection [i.e., mastery].

An Inaugural Discourse on Medical Education. [Delivered at the opening of the Medical College of Ohio, Cincinnati, Ohio, November 11.] Cincinnati: Looker, Palmer, and Reynolds, 1820.

Reader Reflection

1. *This is one of the early presentations that medicine is art form involving application of the precepts of science to the care of the patient. What does it mean to combine the science and art in the practice of medicine?*
2. *How can the knowledge of the "ancients" or "literature" help the aspiring physician to become an artist in caring for a patient? Or in your field of endeavor?*

4.29 Lifelong Learning

You have at an early period manifested a conviction, that knowledge can only be acquired by application. Let me exhort you to follow ardently in the suggestions of this conviction, for a professional man can never neglect them with impunity. When you leave the medical school your studies are merely begun. The germ of your future professional knowledge yet a tender seedling, which neglected by you must inevitably parish. Watch over it then unceasingly—foster it with tenderness—supply with liberality and you will elevate it in time to a magnificent tree. Its balmy exhalations will diffuse health and comfort among the wretched victims of disease;—the golden fruit of its wide spreading branches will supply your numerous wants, and, in the shade of its ever green foliage you will glide serenely down the vale of declining life. Your studies ought not therefore to terminate with your residence in college. They should be continued diligently through all the engagements, the vicissitudes, and the trials of after life.

"Valedictory Address to the Class at Lexington in the Transylvania University, 1818." Daniel Drake Collection, Box 2, Folder 1. Henry R. Winkler Center for the History of the Health Professions, Donald Harrison Health Sciences Library, University of Cincinnati.

Reader Reflection

1. *What seeds of knowledge and learning were sown in your formal schooling that will need to be nourished and applied to see them grow and bear fruit?*
2. *What new knowledge areas would you like to pursue? How will becoming a lifelong learner be beneficial to your career?*

Physician

"A Learned and Distinguished Physician"

"I had great confidence in his professional acumen; I saw enough of him in the sick chamber to satisfy me that he had a most minute and thorough knowledge of disease, and of the application of remedial [medical] agents. There was no one whom I would rather have trusted in my own case, or in that of a member of my family."
—Samuel Gross, MD, *A Discourse on the Life, Character, and Services of Daniel Drake, M.D.*

5.1   *Disease: The Foe in the Battle*

5.2   *Recognize the Distress That Disease Brings and Dispense Hope*

5.3   *Being a Physician: Scientific Treatment and Caring*

5.4   *A Physician Is a Member of the Community*

5.5   *The Role of the Medical Profession in Society*

5.6   *A Physician Must Have a Comprehensive Understanding of the Nature of Man*

5.7   *Recognize the Interaction between the Mind and Body*

5.8   *Successful Physicians Learn What It Means to Be a Human Being*

5.9   *The Determinants of Health and Disease in the Interior Valley*

5.10 *The Moral Dimension of Being a Physician*

5.11 *The Positive Power of Honorable Ambition*

5.12 *Fight against Descending into Self-Interest*

5.13 *Learn to Scrutinize and Don't Accept "Facts" on Blind Faith*

5.14 *Success in Science Requires Patience and Persistence*

5.15 *Recognize How Difficult Comprehending and Practicing Medicine Is*

5.16 *Forecasting a Young Physician's Future*

5.17 *Habits Essential for Improving in Practice*

5.18   *Medical Practice Requires Replenishing Your Knowledge*

5.19   *Read the Works of the Masters in the First Years of Practice*

5.20   *Developing a Physician's Style and Reputation*

5.21   *How a Person Is Shaped by His "Probationary Period"*

5.22   *Don't Make Premature Conclusions about a Case*

5.23   *The First Medical Case Report from Cincinnati*

5.24   *Learning How to Keep Healthy*

5.25   *The Calamitous Effects of Intemperance*

5.26   *Be Able to Describe the Natural History of a Disease: Milk Sickness*

5.27   *A Case of Depression Beginning with Burn Trauma and Ending with Outdoor Exercise*

5.28   *Description of Post-traumatic Neuralgia Following a Severe Burn*

5.29   *Nature Therapy*

5.30   *First Report of the Ohio Lunatic Asylum*

5.31   *Diagnosing and Predicting the Cholera Epidemic*

5.32   *Analyzing Data to Reach a Valid Conclusion*

5.33   *Factors in the Patient's Predisposition Shape the "Host Response"*

5.34   *The Three-Year Experience of Cholera in Cincinnati and Lessons Learned This Far*

5.35   *Thoughts on How Medicines Work and Opium as a Selected Example*

5.36   *Public Health While Traveling on the Rivers: Three Recommendations*

5.37   *An Advocate for Vaccination*

5.38   *Causes of Professional Quarrels*

5.39   *The Compensation of Physicians*

5.40   *Improve Upon Your Own Work for Future Generations*

Chapter Five

— *Drake was a pioneer in the medical field and in Cincinnati. In 1800 he became the first medical student in Cincinnati, and four years later he was the first Cincinnati student to receive a medical diploma.*

— *Twelve years after earning his diploma, Drake graduated from the University of Pennsylvania in 1816, becoming the first medical student from Cincinnati to graduate from a medical school.*

— *He helped to expand the medical field in Ohio and Kentucky. In 1826 he established the Cincinnati Eye Infirmary, making him the first MD west of the Alleghenies to devote attention to eye disorder.*

— *Recognizing the importance of medical discussion and community, Drake founded the First District Medical Society in Cincinnati in 1812. He was active in organized medicine his entire career and served as a founding member of the American Medical Association in 1847.*

▨ AUTHOR INTRODUCTION

The practice of medicine in Drake's time was rooted in the prescientific theories of medicine popular in the late 1700s, with limited knowledge of disease mechanisms and even less of effective treatments. Some treatments popularized by individual physicians had no scientific basis. Medical journals were still in their infancy and no medical schools existed in Cincinnati when Drake was apprenticed for four years to Dr. William Goforth. Drake later became a student of Dr. Benjamin Rush in Philadelphia who advocated and taught the "heroic depletion theory," an aggressive regimen of bloodletting, purgatives (e.g., calomel—mercury-based cathartics), and sweating to shock the body back into health after a humoral imbalance. This was the basis of Drake's medical treatments. Medicine was still seeking to build its scientific foundations. The movement toward understanding localized pathology and associating that pathology to the cause of specific symptoms and physical signs, which began in France in the early 1800s, was yet to shape and influence American medicine.

The approach to learning about disease in practice for Drake was to develop his powers of observation and description and study the natural history of the disease and its response to different treatments. This naturalist's approach is what he learned as a student in Philadelphia, and he utilized this approach his entire career. Drake advised young physicians to develop their system of medicine, that is, a comprehensive understanding of what causes disease, and to recognize the limitations of what physicians can do. His understanding of human beings and what causes disease was broad. He recognized that the mental state of the patient or family and the interaction of the mind and body were part of the illness experience and were to be addressed in treating patients. Physicians primarily attended patients in their homes and would remain present in the setting of serious and grave illness. Drake witnessed the distress that illness brings to the patient and family, and he felt it was the physician's responsibility to be serene, project confidence, and offer hope. For him this was the basis of being an effective physician. The physician played an important role in the community, and he recognized that virtuous character was an important asset to the physician.

Over the course of his career he continued to create his own model for health and disease, which was very progressive. He recognized that diseases were common to a specific topography and climate and were often due to specific habits of diet, occupation, family, and social factors. This sort of knowledge was foundational for the physician as a starting point for diagnosis. He stressed the importance of collecting accurate data and then analyzing and interpreting the data, recognizing that in the absence of a scientific method of study, most interpretations generated hypotheses and unproven explanations. This is seen in his studies of milk sickness and cholera and in his two-volume *Systematic Treatise on the Principal Diseases of the Interior Valley of North America*.

His legacy as a physician includes his setting high standards for the profession, his emphasis on the physician's character, his inclusion of public health, and finally his comprehensive model for the determinants of health and disease in a community. These contributions remain relevant for every generation.

✖ 5.1 Disease: The Foe in the Battle

Disease is a foe which invades us in as many forms as Proteus could assume. It is the great enemy of all enterprise and improvement: the sedative which paralyzes every faculty and passion: the poison which deranges every mental operation: the opposing power of patriotism, philanthropy, and ambition—relaxing the arm of industry, subverting the schemes of benevolence, and extinguishing the lights of genius, to lead him captive through the mazes of error and dullness. It may be likened to the dark cloud which intercepts the sun beams till the germinating corn perishes in the earth; or the baleful mist that spreads mildew over the ripening harvest;—nay, its ravages are terrible as the volcano which breaks up the foundations of a country; prostrating as the tempest that lays waste its cultivated surface; overwhelming as the inundation which buries up its monuments, and "completes the work of devastation and ruin."

The struggle of the medical profession with this fell power, can only be compared to the holy but interminable contest of truth with error and falsehood; or the glorious warfare that liberty maintains against the black empire of despotism:— the magazines of science supply the shield and armour, philanthropy inspires the heroism, and the life of man is the prize of victory.

An Inaugural Discourse on Medical Education. [Delivered at the opening of the Medical College of Ohio, Cincinnati, Ohio. November 11.] Cincinnati: Looker, Palmer, and Reynolds, 1820. 31.

Reader Reflection

1. *Disease is part of the human condition with far-reaching effects shaping the course of culture. Do you take note on the epic battles that are playing out in your life and community? Are you engaged as well? How does working in collaboration with others help with such battles?*

2. *What is the burden of disease in your community? What segments of the population are prevented from reaching their potential due to the presence of disease?*

✖ 5.2 Recognize the Distress That Disease Brings and Dispense Hope

I shall not dwell exclusively on the pains and sufferings of the sick; but call your attention, likewise, to the various distresses of which disease is the fruitful parent.

To estimate these, we must have approached its unfortunate subjects, and mingled with those who hung in anxiety and anguish over the sick bed. The united agonies of mind and body experienced, even by a disgusting victim of prodigality and vice, affect us so sensibly that we cannot but desire his recovery, and feel inclined to unite with him in sentiments of gratitude to the physician who restores him to health, and perhaps to reformation and happiness. But what is there in the maladies of an insulated wretch to excite our pity, in comparison with the sufferings of the unfortunate, the useful and the good?...

But the apprehensions of society for the fate of a great and good man in disease sink into insignificance when compared with the forebodings and anguish of his friends and family. Who has ever cast his eye upon the death-bed of such a man, without the conviction that it is a scene of the deepest anguish? Who has, at any time, gazed on the sad spectacle of weeping relatives, supplicating friends, and distracted children, and not been suddenly pervaded with horror? Who has ever contemplated the affectionate wife, immovably fixed at the head of her expiring husband, absorbed in unutterable grief, and silently rent with pangs of sorrow; and not turned in sympathetic dismay towards that profession, upon which, in these hours of emergency and distraction, the good as well as the bad, the wise as well as the foolish, are compelled to rely for hope and relief? When such a man is the prize, to rescue him from the grasp of death, and dissipate the portentous gloom that hangs over his family and friends, by the light of his renovated eye, is one of the happiest efforts of the medical profession. But although among the happiest, it is not the noblest triumph of medicine. There are periods of epidemic disease, in which the King of Terrors envelopes society in a pestilential cloud; when the salutation of the morning is not, who has expired, but who has survived through the night; when the stillness of our highways is interrupted only by the solemn rumblings of the hearse, and the silence of our apartments unbroken, except by the groans of the dying, and the more melancholy wailings of those who watch around; when Despair spreads her lurid mantle over the portals of every habitation; and Horror infuses his chilling influence into every vein, till the stoutest hearts are appalled; when Calamity sways his iron sceptre, and Terror, like a whirlwind, breaks asunder the bonds of society, and involves its members in anarchy and desolation:—then it is, when the ties of consanguinity and love have been dissolved, till the mother abandons her infected son, and the husband deserts his dying wife,—at this awful crisis, the good physician arises in a panoply of knowledge, as the champion of humanity. Deeply impressed with the sacred duties of his office, and nobly animated to their faithful performance, he sustains an aspect of serenity and confidence, and sublimely goes forth, like a ministering angel, to dispense health and hope and happiness.

An Inaugural Discourse on Medical Education. [Delivered at the opening of the Medical College of Ohio, Cincinnati, Ohio. November 11.] Cincinnati: Looker, Palmer, and Reynolds, 1820. 25–28.

READER REFLECTION

1. *Drake had personally lost a daughter (Harriet, eleven months) and son (John, nearly three years) at the time when these remarks were shared. He had firsthand experience of the emotional impact of disease on the patient and family. It is this deep awareness that motivated him to care and try to restore the sick person back to health. What personal motivation drives you in your work? Does your motivation come from your "character"? If not, from where did it originate?*

2. *Reflect upon the duties of the physician in caring for both patient and family.*

✠ 5.3 BEING A PHYSICIAN: SCIENTIFIC TREATMENT AND CARING

There is, gentlemen, no profession on earth that calls so loudly for benevolence in its professors as our own. This benevolence has two great modes of action, or rather two objects, to heal the sick man and soothe him while the cure is advancing. I am sorry to say that there are two kinds of benevolent physicians, the physician of one kind contents himself with the accomplishment of the cure, and is a petty tyrant throughout its progress, the other sums up his duty, in those kind attentions which soothe the feelings of the patient, comparatively regard less of the great end of medical duty. One with a rude and unfeeling grasp rescues the victim from death, the other lets him go, but kindly and industriously constructs a little railway for his ease and comfort—pours out upon him many tender expressions, beguiles him with flattering speeches and politely bows him into the grave. *I need not tell you gentlemen that each of these characters is defective. The humanity of the physician should both soothe and save.*

"The Formation of Professional Character" [1835]. In *Frontiersman of the Mind,* edited by Charles D. Aring. Cincinnati: History of the Health Sciences Library and Museum, University of Cincinnati, 1985.

Reader Reflection

1. *Drake's approach to the patient included both the scientific treatments of his day (save) and responding to the emotional needs of the patient (soothe). He is saying here that doctoring requires both. Discuss why both are needed in the care of the patient.*
2. *What is the role of the placebo in the current practice of medicine?*

☒ 5.4 A Physician Is a Member of the Community

Medicine is a physical science, but a social profession. What skeletons are to the comparative anatomist, and plants to the botanist, people in health and disease are to the physician. Both his elementary studies and his after duties are prosecuted in their midst, and can be pursued no where else. He maybe in feeling a cynic, or in taste a recluse, but, practically, he must be ever present among the masses, acting and being re-acted on by them. Thus, *per necessitatem*, he is made a member of the community in which he follows his vocation, and becomes more or less colored by its characteristic dyes.

"Early Physicians, Scenery, and Society of Cincinnati." *Discourses Delivered by Appointment before the Cincinnati Medical Library Association.* Cincinnati: Moore and Anderson, 1852. 49.

Reader Reflection

1. *Medicine as a social profession is rooted in the community. Study the community as patient. What are the community diagnoses?*
2. *How is your community shaping and forming you as you practice? Is this true of other professions too?*

☒ 5.5 The Role of the Medical Profession in Society

When a serious disease attacks an only son, on the threshold of manhood, and threatens the sudden extinction of genius and enterprise; or, when it fixes on a favorite daughter, in the midst of bloom and beauty, while every virtue is germinating in her youthful bosom, and the first fruits of taste and intelligence afford full sustenance to future hope—to what can we compare the agony and consternation of the afflicted parents? Or what language could express their gratitude to him who should preserve such beloved objects from a premature grave? To accomplish this deliverance would be an enviable achievement; but a nobler triumph attends the conquest of the Tyrant, when his vengeful arrows are fixed on manhood in the zenith of its splendor. Men of genius and beneficence are the brightest luminaries of the moral firmament: the choicest gifts of bounteous Heaven to our benighted race. They were the authors and architects of society; they decoyed the hunter out of the wilderness and weaned him from the chase; encircled him with the arts and sciences; inspired him with new and nobler propensities, and continue to furnish him with the means of gratification and happiness. In their preservation and prosperity then we should feel a deep and living interest. When they are assailed by disease, the very pillars of society are menaced with destruction; and their expiring struggles spread convulsion and disorder throughout whole communities. When a catastrophe of this kind impends; when our divines, philosophers, and statesmen; our artisans, physicians, advocates, professors, and philanthropists, are selected as the victims of disease; when the fountains of benefaction begin to pour forth troubled waters, and we are even threatened with a diminished supply of these, where do we then look for relief, or on what can we rely but the medical profession?

An Inaugural Discourse on Medical Education. [Delivered at the opening of the Medical College of Ohio, Cincinnati, Ohio. November 11.] Cincinnati: Looker, Palmer, and Reynolds, 1820. 26.

READER REFLECTION
1. *The medical profession cares for all people living in a community. Should physicians who have the responsibility of caring for leaders and benefactors of a community feel a special privilege and weight in seeking to preserve their health and restore them from sickness? It is a contribution to the community to keep our leaders well.*
2. *Consider why a community has an interest in securing a competent healthcare workforce.*

▨ 5.6 A Physician Must Have a Comprehensive Understanding of the Nature of Man

Man, being a compound of mind and body, can only be understood by observing and studying both, for they act and re-act upon each other. In the successive periods of life, in different individuals, and in various grades of civilization, the relative power of the mind upon the body, and the body upon the mind, is different. Thus, in the civilized and intellectual state, the mind exercises great power over the body, than in the savage state; and the mind of a philosopher, or a Christian, governs the desires of his body more effectually, than the mind of an ignorant or wicked person controls his appetites; and, finally, the mind of an adult rules over his bodily wants, with greater success than the mind of a child. In the tender stages of infancy, the reasoning powers and the moral sentiments are but little developed, and the corporeal appetites and desires are strong. The reason is obvious. The body must be built up, and hence the appetite for food and the pleasures of indulgence are great, sometimes almost insatiable. The impatience of labor is quick, because its industry can seldom be turned to good account, and its limbs are soon fatigued, while they are growing; its natural repugnance to close or long continued confinement is equally strong, for fresh air and unrestrained exercise are requisite to the proper maintenance of health; its curiosity for wandering among new objects is intense, and indispensable to its growth; finally, its love of play and of pleasure is almost indomitable; because on the plan of nature, no responsibility in regard to the future rests upon it; and if it had not a desire for play, it would not take the necessary exercise, nor acquire the proper use and discipline of its limbs. Thus, almost all the pains and pleasures of infancy and youth, connect themselves with the body. The gratification of the physical and material part is the great object; that which answers to the wants and desires of the body, and for the present moment. Its enjoyments are physical—its sufferings are physical; and, when they extend to the mind, it is because something which administered to the pleasures of the sense has been withheld, or applied in such manner as to mortify the few feelings and sentiments of the soul, which, at an early period, are in a state of susceptibility.

"Discipline: Discourse on the Philosophy of Family, School, and College Discipline." *Transactions of the Fourth Annual Meeting of the Western Literary Institute and College of Professional Teachers.* [Held in Cincinnati October 1834.] Cincinnati: Josiah Drake Publisher, 1835. 36, 37.

Reader Reflection

1. *"In successive periods of life, in different individuals, and in various grades of civilization, the relative power of the mind upon the body, and the body upon the mind, is different." How do you think the mind influences the body and the body influences the mind? Any personal examples?*
2. *Give an example of the mind-body interaction in yourself that you would like to gain better control of mind over body.*

5.7 Recognize the Interaction between the Mind and Body

We have often observed with regret, that many physicians are more ignorant of the philosophy of the mind, than of anything else connected with the human constitution; and that many of them have not even perceived the necessity of studying the laws of man's nobler part. All this is wrong. The reciprocal influence of the mind and body is a fact which should never be forgotten by the physician; and, indeed, it is not; but how few have made it a study! How few have had a realizing sense of its importance! Every enlightened and experienced physician has seen diseases produced by mental emotion, protracted by the same cause in spite of his physical remedies, or, finally removed by the rise of an opposite emotion. But it is in the study and treatment of the innumerable varieties of mental aberration that the value of this branch of physiological science appears in its greatest magnitude; and no practitioner should ever approach the unfortunate subject of one of these alienations, without a familiar acquaintance with the principles of the philosophy of the mind as well as the body. Finally there is still another and very different reason for cultivating intellectual philosophy. Physicians are the teachers of medical students, and to teach successfully, they must be well acquainted with this branch of science.

"Lectures on Mental Philosophy of Students of Medicine." *Western Journal of the Medical and Physical Sciences Cincinnati* 10 (1836): 324.

Reader Reflection

1. *"Mental Philosophy" was the term applied to the psychological dimension in Drake's time. The field was not yet defined. Despite this lack of knowledge his clinical experience taught him how important mind-body interactions influence the illness experience of the patient where symptoms were protracted or improved by the patient's emotional state. How does a physician identify a mind-body interaction that is influencing the disease/illness experience in the patient? What can the physician do to impact the patient's mind-body interaction in a positive way?*

5.8 Successful Physicians Learn What It Means to Be a Human Being

The reason that so many branches of human knowledge unite in the medical profession is to be found in the varied and intimate relations of man with all the objects and operations of nature, all the works of art, and all the events of society and the world. It is these extended connections that make him under God, its governor; that constitute him the greatest, not less the latest, of its organized beings. In his perfect development he lives, and feels, and thinks, and acts, amid things and movements as countless in number as the leaves of our summer woods—as diversified in aspect as their forms and autumnal tints. The oak, on the summit of the hill, has a relation only to the soil, the winds, the rain, and the thunderbolt, which may at last rive it asunder. The flower, which blooms beneath its wide-spreading branches, is sustained by the evening and morning dew, the shower, and the sun; and having these, it sends forth it fragrance for a season, and dies a natural death. The wild deer of our forest crop the natural herbage, escape from the wolf, and lie down in their grassy lair, until age puts an end to an existence more simple than that of any human being. The passenger pigeon leaves the south, as the heat of summer arises, spends a season in the north, rears it young, and returns to the place of departure. Its relations are with food, and water, and temperature, and the air by which it performs its migrations. The dwellers in the deep, from the whale to the coral insect, have relations to the water in which they live, and to each other, on which, in part, they feed, and to these they are confined. Far different from all these limited connections and dependencies are those which man sustains with other portions of the creation. His instincts and his wants, corporeal, intellectual, and moral, lead him into all climates. In the south he lodges under the boughs of trees, in the north in huts built of compacted snow, and on the swampy banks of lakes and rivers he drives down piles on which to support his dwellings. Go into the sandy desert, and there you find his tents; turn your eyes to the bleak mountain-top, and there you see his cabin embosomed in the cloud; look upon the ocean, and you behold it white with canvas of his floating habitations, driven to and fro by the tempest. On the broad continents he cuts down, and burns or applies to his own use, the mightiest forests; his plowshare annihilates the natural herbage, and his sagacity and toil replace it with productions more to his taste, or better suited to his wants; in one region he lives solitary, and gives full play to all his desires and fancies; in another he struggles through the conflicting masses of a city population, where he invents new modes of industry; dooms himself to a confined and unventilated room, or a dark and damp cellar; passes much of every day in some constrained posture; breathes an atmosphere impregnated with irritating dust, or poisonous gases; watches his rivals, and seeks to wrap himself up from their scrutiny; labors to outstrip them in the career of mingled ambition and avarice; concocts schemes for their defeat, or his own advancement; delivers himself over to midnight studies, or gluts his pampered appetites with meats and drinks, drawn from the abounding storehouses of every kind. He founds and conducts institutions of benevolence, literature, and science; devises enterprises which demand concert of action, adventures on gigantic projects the most visionary; and grasps riches, with power and luxury which they bestow, or involves himself and others in hopeless ruin.

When we look into man's organization, organism, and internal functions—his capacities of body—his faculties of mind—and the emotions and desires of his heart—we find a fullness, variety, and perfection—a complexity—a quickness of irritability and a delicacy of feeling, nowhere else to be found in the world of organized nature; fitting him admirably for the position he occupies in the world; but, at the same time rendering him vulnerable to a thousand influences. If he act on all around, everything around reacts on him. If he shape and fashion them to his liking, these, in turn, modify his organization, impress on him peculiarities of constitution—develop one organ into excessive dimensions, and arrest the growth of another—exalt this sensibility, and depress that—break up the equilibrium of his vital functions, and derange his system with a greater variety of diseases, than are found in the whole kingdom of organized nature, of which he is at once the monarch and the victim.

Such, young gentlemen, is the being whose diseases you will be called upon to prevent and heal. To accomplish the former, you must inquire into the action all the influences, material and mental, to which he may be subjected, and either withdraw him from them, or fortify his constitution against their deleterious impress. But how can you do this, without that power which knowledge bestows? How can you detect the sinister agency of the water that he drinks—or the food he eats—or the soil which he tills—or the shop in which he labors—or the climate which he breathes—or the passion by which he is consuming away—unless you have studied their nature, and know the relations which they bear to his constitution of body and mind? But, you will be called upon, still oftener, to cure, than prevent his diseases; and how can you perform that part of your mission, without a thorough and diversified knowledge, of the effects of the multitude of agents, which exert their influence on his constitution? In proportion to this knowledge, will be the richness of your resources—according to your sagacity and sound judgment, will be your success in application.

An Introductory Lecture, at the Opening of the Thirtieth Session of the Medical College of Ohio. Cincinnati: Morgan and Overend Printers, 1849. 6–7.

READER REFLECTION

1. *Drake was a systems thinker—taking a holistic view to analyze, focusing on how the constituent parts interrelate to cause or influence each other. How does a person become good at thinking systemically?*

2. *Every career has this sort of knowledge that is acquired after formal education. Imagine a young student in your field asks you what knowledge you learned after your formal education that has been the most important to your success. What would you say?*

3. *How important is systems thinking to be successful in your career? In your field try applying systems thinking to understand causality and prediction.*

✖ 5.9 THE DETERMINANTS OF HEALTH AND DISEASE IN THE INTERIOR VALLEY

The Interior Valley, or deeply depressed, intermountain plane of North America, has been already announced as the region to which this work relates. Great valleys have both alpine and marine borders, and the medical historian should comprehend them in his researches. Faithful to this duty, and adopting a hydrographical method, I have ascended our streams to their mountain sources, or descended them to the sea, at points exceedingly distant from each other. The vast extent of this field of inquiry would, at first view, seem to be a great disadvantage, but it is, in fact, highly favorable to the development of results; as it enables us to trace a disease, in continuity, from its point of greatest prevalence, to its disappearance under new physical or moral or social conditions.

To these conditions I wish now to direct the attention of the reader. When they are subjected to a first analysis, we find them resolved into three principal groups. The first comprehends all that belong to the earth, considered in the composition and mechanical arrangement of it superficial strata, the quality of its soil, and the amount, distribution, and quality of its waters: these are the telluric or geological influences. Second comprises all that belong to the atmosphere, and its mechanical action, sensible qualities, and adventitious impregnations: which make the climactic or meteorological influences. To the third belongs whatever appertains to society, considered in reference to national physiology, density of population, diet, drinks, clothing, occupations, amusements, intellectual cultivation, and moral improvement: in which are embraced the social and physiological influences.

If in countries their geological, hydrographical, topographical, climactic, social, and physiological conditions were nearly the same, of course their medical histories would be much alike; but if they different widely in one or several of these conditions, the corresponding diversity would appear in the respective histories of all the diseases, which admit of modification from causes referable to those [categories].

Systematic Treatise, Historical, Etiological, and Practical, on the Principal Diseases of the Interior Valley of North America as They Appear in the Caucasian, African, Indian, and Esquimaux Varieties of Its Population. Cincinnati: Winthrop B. Smith & Co., 1850. 1: 2–3.

Reader Reflection

1. *From his long career Drake identified the determinants of health and disease working in the Interior Valley: geological, hydrological, climatological (physical determinant), the physiological (now including genetics and the body's response), the moral (cultural), and the social (diet, clothing, occupation, amusements). This was highly original and presaged by nearly 150 years a working model of health and disease in place today. How can the study of epidemiology inform your practice?*

2. *How does your understanding of the determinants of health shape your approach to understanding the burden of disease in your community? In the individual patient?*

3. *Many of these determinants are outside the work of a physician and are shaped by public policy. Drake was involved in public health efforts. What public health problems exist in your county?*

5.10 The Moral Dimension of Being a Physician

How important it is that the physician should be a conscientious man, who has other motives for investigating the principles of the profession, than the fear of having his ignorance detected and exposed! He should shrink with horror from the idea of prescribing on false premises, or by loose and un-philosophical analogies. He should recollect that human life is at stake; that a human being in extremity is confided to his skill and honor; and that an ignorant or presumptuous stroke of his pen may translate that confiding fellow creature—perhaps his bosom friend—from time to eternity, to confront him with damning testimony on the day of final retribution. Although such practice is not legally felonious, it deserves unqualified denunciation; for in a moral view, where lies the line of distinction between criminal prescriptions and those which prove fatal, through criminal ignorance of their authors? I say criminal *ignorance*, for although, in the abstract, there is no criminality in being unacquainted with the truth, yet, in the practice of medicine, to be ignorant of facts and principles, which lie within the grasp of common minds under common opportunities, and still to undertake that, which they, only, who are acquainted with these facts can accomplish, is to forget the divine maxim of doing to others as we would be done unto; and, literally to wage war upon human life; not in malice prepense [intentional] towards any individual, but with the senseless and fatal impartiality of an epidemic disease.

"Causes of Error in the Medical and Physical Sciences." In *Practical Essays on Medical Education and the Medical Profession in the United States.* Cincinnati: Roff & Young, 1832. 88.

Reader Reflection

1. *What is the motivation in your profession/in medicine to keep knowledge up to date? Are there safeguards to prevent the ills Drake describes from happening?*
2. *What are other professions in addition to medicine where ignorance can cause great harm?*
3. *Discuss: Is keeping current with the progress of knowledge foundational to a person's enduring legacy?*

5.11 The Positive Power of Honorable Ambition

In the cultivation and practice of science, which is imperfect and speculative, no principle of action is so powerful as ambition.... The lover of truth, who is content with its acquisition, has less enjoyment than he who superadds useful application to accurate attainment; and of all the original principles of our nature, the desire of honorable fame is not only most beneficial to the world, but one of the most ennobling to the soul which it animates.

We must not confound this ambition with either pride or vanity. The former preserves us from little actions, but never impels us to great—the latter contents itself with vulgar admiration, and incites us to those performances only which bring immediate applause. Pride looks to society for no reward, either present or prospective; vanity undertakes nothing on trust—is not willing to rely on posterity for payment—exacts daily returns from the surrounding multitude, and slakes its thirst with draughts of flattery and adulation. Ambition, in itself, has no element either good or bad. It works as a mere animating principle; and rouses us to deeds of desperation and death, or schemes of beneficence and life, according to the moral sense and the objects of each individual. When it subjugates the heart, and arrays itself in the armor of misanthropy, it delights in nothing, but new advances over a terrified and prostate world; but subordinate to the heart, it becomes the bright sun of society, and cheers and vivifies whatever its beams may fall upon. Such is the ambition, which should glow in the bosom of every physician; he would then see no mountain too lofty to be scaled, nor so overhung with murky vapours, that he could not discern the clear and beautiful sky that stretches out beyond its summits. Warmed by love for mankind, enamoured of his profession and animated by the hope of rising higher than all who had trodden its rugged steeps before him, he would move on his upward march, with never a tiring step. Not too proud to employ every honorable means, however humble; nor so vain as to loiter, by the way to catch the siren sounds of popular applause, he would see and think and dream of nothing, but the grandeur which surrounds the objects that allured him on. He would suppose all the time, that these being attained, he might sit down in the midst of them, and give himself up to enjoyment. But the man of true ambition never stops to revel in the camp of victory. He delights in action and anticipation, and looks with rapture from his new elevation, at the distant and loftier pinnacles, which till then were hidden from his view. Finally, the physician of honorable ambition has no quiet sleep, while any are before him. He would not keep them back, but advance himself—he does not regard them with envy, but emulation. He even extends to them his respect, but this requires no ordinary effort, and the magnanimity of his character is seen in the candor with which he can bring himself to view their merits, and identify their fame with the glory of his profession.

"Causes of Error in the Medical and Physical Sciences." In *Practical Essays on Medical Education and the Medical Profession in the United States.* Cincinnati: Roff & Young, 1832. 83–85.

Reader Reflection

1. *How strong is ambition working in you as an animating principle for your life goals?*
2. *Are there other good motivations for success besides personal ambition?*
3. *Ambition can have a negative connotation, but how does Drake describe "honorable ambition" as a positive? How is this different from pride or vanity?*

⊠ 5.12 Fight against Descending into Self-Interest

The love of truth, although an original principle of human nature, has various degrees of native energy; and from the operation of several causes, may decline, till we come to look upon error with complacency, and at last not only tolerate but publish falsehood. Very few principles of our nature, are, indeed, beset with so many causes of corruption. I will name but two—self-interest and self-love. The combined influence of these on the love and practice of truth, in morals and society at large, is seen and admitted by all; and it is equally great in the medical sciences, where, although less deprecated, it is perhaps still more mischievous....

As physicians and surgeons, when we expect to receive patronage, less in the proportion of our true knowledge than of our plausibility, that the temptation to deceive, both ourselves and others, acquires an irresistible and frightful energy. As the naturalists find it necessary to supply the analogy, the lost parts of a Mammoth skeleton, before it can satisfy vulgar curiosity, so physicians feel the importance of presenting an aspect of perfect knowledge, when they would acquire public confidence. This imposture, not often detected, still more seldom frowned upon, by the hoodwinked community, whose unreasonable demands have invited it; and, as impunity promotes the repetition of the crime, one imposition follows another, till the love of truth falls gradually into ruins; and the heart once honest and open becomes at last polluted with the principles of criminal selfishness. The guileless lineaments of unsophisticated nature are now exchanged for the studied imitations of art; and the question no longer is, what does truth require, but what will best administer to the insatiable cravings of self-interest, and where lie the moral limits which cannot be overstepped, without injury of reputation? Mark the physician who has thus degenerated, and you will no longer perceive in him any sacred veneration for professional truth.

"Causes of Error in the Medical and Physical Sciences." In *Practical Essays on Medical Education and the Medical Profession in the United States.* Cincinnati: Roff & Young, 1832. 80–81.

Reader Reflection

1. *How does self-interest undermine the practice of medicine—the care of the patient?*
2. *What does it say about a physician who moves from altruism to self-interest?*

✖ 5.13 Learn to Scrutinize and Don't Accept "Facts" on Blind Faith

In all ages, the majority of practitioners have not given themselves the trouble of observing and thinking, but eschewing the investigation of principles, have been contented with adopting the conclusions of those whom they regard as eminent. This doubtless will be the case, as it is easier to walk in the footsteps of a guide than to strike out a new path or even to correct his aberrations. Every distinguished man has his adherents, and when they have once assumed that character they seldom desert either him or his principles. Their successors of the next generation may worship at some other shrine,—a new star ascendant may blaze the zenith—but the old idolaters will in general prefer to keep their gaze upon that which dazzled them in youth. Thus, it is the multitude—the great commonality—who spread and perpetuate the errors of the genius. Their blind devotion is at variance with the spirit of improvement and reform. They are more obedient to the authority of names long venerated, than to facts. They are personal partisans, jealous of the fame of their *Palinurus* [a guide or navigator in Roman mythology], and proud of their fealty, and fetters. Such being the undeniable reality, it is important to scrutinize the opinions and *dicta* of those who are rising into distinction, or whose fame is gradually spreading over the world; that the errors mixed up with the truths they develop may not be implicitly adopted.

"Observations on Some of the Uses and Abuses of Purgatives." *Western Journal of the Medical and Physical Sciences* 7 (1833): 32–42.

Reader Reflection

1. *Devotion to a tradition is "at variance with the spirit of improvement and reform." How common is blind devotion to tradition in your organization/in the practice of medicine? What is the best way of managing it?*

✖ 5.14 Success in Science Requires Patience and Persistence

The highest eulogy that could be pronounced upon patience in research is that it constitutes the great secret of that success, which men of inferior talent so often attain. It *must*, therefore, be a powerful auxiliary, and why should any man reject its assistance? To say that strength of intellect can render it unnecessary is not true....

In his own elevated sphere, the ablest philosopher will find patience essential to the development of truth. Nature is not an oracle of Delphi, to be bribed or flattered into responses. Her severe majesty requires that she should be interrogated patiently, and listened to with meekness; and even when thus besought, her replies may not always be prompt and explicit as we could desire; but they will neither be interested nor erroneous....

Our proper business, then, is the study of material objects, and these must be examined by our organs of sense, to be rightly understood. If this examination be reluctant and superficial, the results will of course be imperfect. If we come to it in a temper of fastidiousness, and shrink from the necessary exertion, because we may have been unused to manual labor, or some parts of that which should be done are unpleasant or repulsive, we shall seldom grasp the truth. If we suppose, that not having been compelled to labor for subsistence, but, nursed in the lap of wealth and luxury, we may leave the drudgery of science to hands already soiled in the field or hardened in the work shop, we shall, at last, be disappointed in our dearest hopes; and mortified to see those whom habits of toil and application have prepared to vanquish every difficulty, stretch immeasurably beyond us in the race of emulation and professional fame. In the pursuit of physical truth, an examination of the objects of nature is the first and greatest work; and he who brings to it the best manual dexterity, the greatest self-independence, and most untiring industry, with the fullest command of his feelings, in relation to scenes and objects, which are often offensive and sometimes loathsome, will, *ceteris paribus* [with other conditions remaining the same], be successful in his most successful in his researches.... If we read the biography of the greatest men, who have adorned the profession or dignified the ranks of the physical science, we shall find them almost as remarkable for their labors of body as of mind. The former, directed to the objects of their ambition, supplied the pabulum, by which the latter was cherished. Such is the order of nature, and no student or physician, who prizes truth or reputation, should ever depart from it.

"Causes of Error in the Medical and Physical Sciences." In *Practical Essays on Medical Education and the Medical Profession in the United States.* Cincinnati: Roff & Young, 1832. 75–78.

READER REFLECTION

1. *Why is patience needed to be successful in research? What other capacities are needed to be successful in research?*

2. *How would you assess potential for success in your field based on your "labors of body [and] of mind"?*

⚔ 5.15 RECOGNIZE HOW DIFFICULT COMPREHENDING AND PRACTICING MEDICINE IS

A cause of error in the medical and physical sciences is...disproportionate between the strength and grasp of our intellectual faculties, and the number and variety of objects upon which they are exercised.

In styling himself "lord of the creation," man has, perhaps, consulted his pride more than his powers. Certain it is, that he is not less dependent on the other objects of creation, than they are on him. These objects, either animate or inanimate, are, to him, absolutely innumerable—they touch him on every side, and stretch from him indefinitely in all directions. Their relations with him and with each other, are never the same for two successive moments;—for group which now surrounds him no more; while he yet contemplates it, changes of composition and character have taken place, which he could neither foresee or prevent. Even individual objects confound him; and when actually in the focus of his physical or intellectual vision, undergo transformations, which surpass his comprehension, and teach him lessons of wisdom and humility. Suppose that all his observations were correct—would this enable him to arrive at philosophical truth? It would not,—unless those observations were extended to all the individual qualities and relations of every object requiring examination. In constructing a system of science, it is not merely necessary to have no bad materials, but an adequate number of good ones. Ignorance is said to be better than error; but this adage refers chiefly to the condition of the mind in regard to further improvement; for, in establishing a system of science, ignorance and error are, perhaps, equally unpropitious.

Nature, moreover, is not only too unlimited in the number of her objects, but their structure and functions too complicated to be studied without mistake. The very 'clods of the valley' present to the philosopher, in their composition, a problem which he cannot undertake to solve without error,...while his own body—an assemblage of intricate organs, mysteriously united, and harmoniously acting and re-acting on each other, from a principle of motion equally mysteriously, presents him with a case, in which the utmost exertion of his powers of observation and reflection will not secure him false conclusions. If such be the inefficiency of genius, how deplorable must be the failures of imbecility:—let dullness, then inquire with anxiety, and publish doubt and hesitation.

"Causes of Error in the Medical and Physical Sciences." In *Practical Essays on Medical Education and the Medical Profession in the United States.* Cincinnati: Roff & Young, 1832. 69–70.

READER REFLECTION

1. *In any field a person must develop a big picture (in Drake's terms a "system of science") of how that field works—the component parts and how they dynamically relate to each other. What is the big picture for your discipline? What are the fundamental components, and how do they relate to each other?*
2. *Describe a time when you felt like you understood a little piece of the big picture better.*
3. *Discuss why it is difficult, if not impossible, to eliminate mistakes in our work. If this is true about ourselves what attitude should we have toward others?*

5.16 FORECASTING A YOUNG PHYSICIAN'S FUTURE

A diploma constitutes the great object of ambition with every student of medicine. This being acquired, he feels disposed to relax in his efforts; and enjoy his new dignity. In the opinion of his teachers, and, of course, of himself, he is qualified for the practical duties of the profession; and a happy feeling of self-complacency, sometimes of self-sufficiency, springs up. He is no longer a pupil, but a physician— walks on a higher level—is surrounded by new associates—and either turns his thoughts toward new objects, or to none at all.

The length of this period varies with the temper and necessities of each individual. If voluntarily prolonged, the omen is decidedly bad. It indicates a want of ambition, of industry, of conscientiousness, or of the *amor scientia* [love of science]. I am grieved to say, that too many of our young physicians are deficient in one or more of these important elements of future eminence; and through life, prefer to vegetate in the lower walks of the profession, when they might ascend and flourish in the higher regions.

The young man of merit regards a diploma as only one of the series of honors which lie within his grasp. He stops to breathe, but still remembers that he has passed through his novitiate only; and must speedily resume the labors by which alone he can hope to reach the highest honors of the profession. Many desire, even resolve, to be distinguished, but neglect to employ the proper means. Aware of the necessity of study, they intend to recommence it; but put off the day of renewed labor until it is too late. Habits of idleness are formed; the allurements of society establish their fascination; examples of partial or temporary success and acquisition of business, without an attention to studies, unfortunately surround and encourage them; the ignorance and credulity of the world disclose to them the possibility of acquiring, without deserving its confidence; hard study begins to appear less indispensable, and more repulsive; their noble resolves are forgotten—their destiny becomes fixed, and a humble one it is. Such are the course and termination, of a majority of those are put to the study of medicine in the United States.

"Studies, Duties, and Interests of Young Physicians." In *Practical Essays on Medical Education and the Medical Profession in the United States*. Cincinnati: Roff & Young, 1832. 61.

Reader Reflection

1. *What predicts success for young persons who are starting their careers? What does Drake say predicts success for a young physician?*

⬛ 5.17 Habits Essential for Improving in Practice

You may perhaps doubt whether amidst the labors and fatigues of an extensive practice it will be possible to find time for so much professional reading. You have observed that the greater number of physicians neither read nor write on medical subjects, and you will perhaps assert with them that the drudgery of professional life leaves no intervals for those important duties. This is saying that the practice of that profession, which requires above all others a vigorous and inquisitive mind, amply stored with facts and principles and perpetually intent on new acquisitions, is utterly inimical to the application necessary to make them. I hope, gentlemen, you will never subscribe to this absurd and dangerous doctrine. It is not impossible for you to be at once laborious practitioners and diligent students, provided that in the early stages of your career, you providently establish compound habits of business and study. These should never be estranged from each other. Their union is natural and necessary: their separation destructive to all our prospects. It is the divorce of professional reading from medical practice that so often produces a melancholy spectacle of an old physician and respectable man, whose philosophical knowledge in his profession is absolutely less than at the hour when he began to exercise it. There are in the course of every day a number of leisure moments, and these you should seize upon for application to your books. You will perhaps be interrupted by a professional call before you have finished a single page, but let not this discourage you. Return to the sentence that was left unfinished and complete it. Fortify yourselves against the delusion that no improvement can be made in this way; that it is necessary to withdraw from the tumult of business, to situations of retirement and tranquility, before you can read with any advantage. This unfortunate opinion has ruined thousands of our profession, and may justly be regarded as one of the causes which have retarded its progress. It is in your power, suffer me to repeat, gentlemen, to form a habit of reading professional books, in the midst of professional business; and if this habit be once completely established your fortune and your fame are secured:... I hope that each of you will make the experiment, and thus secure the prize of glory, which, in our profession, is the reward of those only, who unite theory with practice, and enlightening and correcting both, by reading, observation, and reflection.

"Valedictory Address to the Class at Lexington in the Transylvania University, 1818." Daniel Drake Collection, Box 2, Folder 1. Henry R. Winkler Center for the History of the Health Professions, Donald Harrison Health Sciences Library, University of Cincinnati.

READER REFLECTION

1. *How does a person develop a habit of reading in the midst of constant interruptions? What system or method is needed?*

2. *Is reading your profession's books foundational to be successful in your profession? If this is true, do you think it is less or more necessary now than in Drake's time?*

3. *Learning in medicine and other careers requires observation, reading, and reflection. Do you agree with Drake that your future "fortune and fame" are secured with these?*

5.18 MEDICAL PRACTICE REQUIRES REPLENISHING YOUR KNOWLEDGE

You are well appraised of the necessity there exists, the literary and professional point of view, of my visiting Philadelphia again. That necessity I find every day to increase. You know no business can be conducted without renovating the capital stock, as it becomes wasted. It is now eight years since I commenced the practice of physic, which is a trade in ideas, and I begin seriously to feel an exhaustion of scientific funds. You'll be surprised that I have not felt it before. In truth I have, but not being able to replenish them, I said but little, being willing, like all others, to support my credit as long as it was practical.

Excerpted from a letter [circa 1813] cited in *The Life of Daniel Drake*, by Edward Mansfield. Cincinnati: Applegate & Co., 1855. 112.

READER REFLECTION

1. *How do you know when you need to go "back to school"?*
2. *As you look ahead what are the steps to achievements in performance and credentials you will need to open the doors for your career?*

✖ 5.19 READ THE WORKS OF THE MASTERS IN THE FIRST YEARS OF PRACTICE

The physician who neglects his studies for the first few years after graduation will seldom resume them. *In many respects, this is one of the most important periods of his whole life.* The omissions of youth may be supplied—those of manhood are fatal to our prospects, in proportion to their number and magnitude.

The young physician is not aware how soon his elementary knowledge—much of which is historical and descriptive, rather than philosophical [scientific]—will fade from his mind, when he ceases to study. That which he possesses can only be retained by new additions. He cannot remain stationary; the moment he ceases to acquire, he loses; and this is true, not merely of professional, but of classical and general knowledge.

Hence, every young physician should devote a stated portion of time to the branches of learning in which engaged or should have engaged his attention, before he began the study of medicine. By doing this he would, if previously well taught, soon make himself an able and accurate scholar; or, having been denied the advantage of early opportunities, he might supply many deficiencies, and save himself from gross illiterateness....

[B]ut no physician should regard his education as in any degree complete, until he has read the writings of most of the great observers, and original geniuses, who have adorned the profession in different ages. He will thus trace up established principles, through all their modifications, to their sources, perhaps in remote antiquity. He will, at every step, amass important but neglected facts. He will be taught how to think. Finally, his mind will be enlarged and liberalized by an acquaintance with the revolutions which the science has undergone.

"Studies, Duties, and Interests of Young Physicians." In *Practical Essays on Medical Education and the Medical Profession in the United States.* Cincinnati: Roff & Young, 1832, 62.

READER REFLECTION

1. *Why are the first years of clinical practice, or when one is beginning one's career, "one of the most important periods of [one's] whole life"?*

2. *What must a young physician or a young person starting his or her career do to complete his or her education? What is the benefit of studying the writings of your professions, "great observers and original geniuses" (i.e., the masters)?*

✳ 5.20 DEVELOPING A PHYSICIAN'S STYLE AND REPUTATION

It is in the first few years after graduation in which a young physician forms his manners, or rather his manner. In no vocation is manner more influential. Many young physicians have acquired popularity by the mere force of manner, while others, of equal or greater professional skill, from the same cause, have never become favorites with the public. For such cases I can offer no infallible recipe. Dignity, tenderness, and modesty would seem to be appropriate elements in the deportment of a young physician, whatever may be their effect on the people. They may not inspire confidence in the vulgar, in comparison with impudence and garrulity; but, sooner or later, their influence will be felt and acknowledged. It must, however, be admitted, that public favor is not always the meed [reward, results] of unexceptionable manners, even when sustained by a competent skill.

In these instances, however there is, generally, in the midst of prevailing excellences, some particular defect. For example, the individual may be deficient in tact; or wanting in attention and earnestness—a defect, which, more than most others, will retard the acquisition of business. Nothing captivates the friends of a sick person so much as an earnest and anxious manner on the part of the physician. None are insensible to such a manner, while many will receive it as a substitute both for skill and social refinement....

A young physician, moreover, is, in general, not qualified for any business but that of his profession; and incurs the risk of pecuniary embarrassment whenever he attempts a vocation to which she has not been educated. And this leads me to warn the young physician against contracting debts and liabilities. The young merchant may contract debts with propriety and advantage. His character for punctuality is part of his capital, and should be used; but the only capital of a young physician is his reputation for professional learning, diligence, and fidelity. On this character he should place his sole reliance. All his effort should be directed to its establishment; and whatever can interfere with this important and difficult object should be studiously avoided.

"Studies, Duties, and Interests of Young Physicians." In *Practical Essays on Medical Education and the Medical Profession in the United States*. Cincinnati: Roff & Young, 1832. 66, 68.

READER REFLECTION

1. *Why is it important for you early in your career to work on your personal style of "deportment" with others? How does a person continually improve this?*
2. *How would attending to this contribute to a person's legacy?*

✖ 5.21 HOW A PERSON IS SHAPED BY HIS "PROBATIONARY PERIOD"

One of the first questions which perplexes a young man after his graduation is the choice of the residence. He should, if possible, place himself within the pale of good, that is, of intelligent society. In any other situation, both his mind and manners will degenerate. His companionship should be with the enlightened and refined of both sexes; for his character is to be formed, and should be modeled after a good examples. It is not important that he should remain permanently in his first locality. He should not leave it, however, until he has passed through a period of probation, and acquired a competent amount of practical knowledge. He may then remove to a more extended theater of action, where he ought to spend his life. If he has commenced within the precincts of such a situation, he should hold on till he acquires public confidence, however slow it may seem to be in coming. Not infrequently this is a protracted period, and abounds in anxieties, hopes and fears, impatience, and hypochondriaism. Under these feelings, the young physician too often resolves on a change of residence; and at the moment, when he is on the eve of acquiring business, transfers himself to another town, where, being a stranger, he is doomed to a second probation. Such removals, several times repeated, have proved fatal to the prospects of many, who, remaining patiently in one situation, would found it productive of all they could desire.

"Studies, Duties, and Interests of Young Physicians." In *Practical Essays on Medical Education and the Medical Profession in the United States*. Cincinnati: Roff & Young, 1832. 67.

Reader Reflection

1. *How does your first "place" shape who you become? Do/did you struggle with impatience and a desire to relocate? Why is/was that?*
2. *Why is this period of starting your career termed the "probationary period"? What milestones occur? Discuss what the probationary period in your field looks like.*

5.22 Don't Make Premature Conclusions about a Case

A cause of error consists in forming conclusions, while we should still be observing. [Physicians] of this intellectual temperament may see deeply, but they look in one direction only; and of course form an opinion before all the facts in relation to the case have been reviewed. They might be compared to the judge who decides on the testimony of one of the parties, unconscious that another waits for an audience. The judgment may be honest, and a correct inference from the facts before him, but still it is wrong. Many of the errors which vitiate the experimental sciences, as well as the affairs of social life, are referable to this head; and as the authors of them are conscious not only of loving truth but think they have investigated them, cling with pertinacity to their conclusions. A singularity exhibited by such persons is, that at different times, they are the honest advocates of opposite opinions. The facts, which at one period were presented to them and led to a particular inference, are forgotten; and, subsequently, those of an adverse tendency are casually offered to their notice, when with equal honesty and promptness, they stand forth as the champions of a contrary doctrine. The fault of this character consists in imperfect and limited suggestion—a sort of intellectual *strabismus* or squinting—by which the field of mental vision is narrowed, and the partial mistaken for the universal. The opinions of such men are entitled to respect for their sincerity, but not to adoption for their soundness. They may be true, but should always assumed erroneous. The proper remedy is a constant recurrence to protracted and comprehensive research; that all the facts in the case may be fully represented in the deduction—when this is realized the judgment is true, and then only.

"Causes of Error in the Medical and Physical Sciences." In Practical Essays on Medical Education and the Medical Profession in the United States. Cincinnati: Roff & Young, 1832. 73–74.

READER REFLECTION

1. A common response to a situation is coming to a conclusion before you know all the facts. Assumptions are made on limited data or intuitive impressions. This can happen not only in making a medical diagnosis, but also in a multitude of human interactions at work, in personal relationships, or with social problems. How does a person prevent this from happening, avoiding "intellectual strabismus"?

▨ 5.23 THE FIRST MEDICAL CASE REPORT FROM CINCINNATI

W.W. age 26 years, with a flat chest, and distant shoulders, was seized in July with a severe cough, and inability to lie with his head and shoulders low. After trying the use of some popular remedies for several days, with no good effect, he applied to me. Finding his skin cool, his pulse low and weak, his thorax entirely free from pain and stricture, and that he had no thirst, and could walk about, I did not at first suspect the existence of inflammation. An emetic and cathartic, with a subsequent use of anodynes, and a plaster of burgundy pitch, were employed without any advantage whatever. In three or four days he was unable to lie down at all. His exemption from pain, and weak pulse continued; but it was determined to bleed him.—About 8 ounces were taken, which exhibited some slight traces of buff [yellowish color]. A blister was in applied to the side. His pulse did not rise, from bleeding, but as he felt rather better, the next day it was repeated to the quantity of 12 ounces. The blood drawn this day was more sizy [thick, viscous]; and after the operation, his pulse rose a little. On the succeeding day he was bled again. The blood exhibited much inflammatory crust, and after the operation his pulse became full, tense, and frequent. His cough continuing, the administration of calomel, with squills [a lily-like plant] and nitre, was now commenced, venesection [blood-letting], to the quantity of 14 or 16 ounces, was continued every day, or every other day, from this time for a week, the pulse beating 120 strokes in a minute, with a great degree of energy. The blood was remarkably cupped and sizy. By the expiration of that time, a salvation came on. No considerable reduction of the pulse followed, but he was able to lie with his head and shoulders lower. Use of the digitalis was then begun. It was given in substance. In three or four days the expected intermissions in the pulse occurred, and it was soon at 60 and 54 in a minute, having sustained an equal reduction in its force and fullness. The half cough became more moderate, expectoration increased, and his amendment was unequivocal. The digitalis has been continued ever since (a period of six months) in such qualities as generally keep his pulse in a state of defective action; he has taken exercise on horseback, and at this time has a good prospect of complete restoration.

Notices Concerning Cincinnati. Cincinnati: John W. Browne and Company, 1810.

Reader Reflection
This case is an example of a patient with probable bronchitis improving in spite of his treatment!
1. *Case reports are an excellent way to learn. Record your observations during the unfolding of a case and note the responses to specific treatments/interventions.*
2. *Consider summarizing a "case" or scenario from your work. Capture the key issues, reflect on possible solutions, and forecast ahead the possible or desired outcomes. Share your insights with a colleague.*

5.24 Learning How to Keep Healthy

From the latter part of December to the 10th or 12th of this month, my dyspepsia increased alarmingly, and I decreased in weight until I was 20 pounds lighter than when I was in my 21st year. I have at length adopted a course of diet, exercise, and regimen, which has produced a promising effect; and, when on the eve of abandoning my profession, and journeying with my family till restored, I have been prevented, and encouraged to trudge forward as usual, by the occurrence of several occurrences of returning health. I have not tasted coffee or tea for six weeks, any kind or variety of bread for nearly 5. I cannot drink wine, Brandy, cider, beer, or Porter; and my only beverage is a tablespoonful of old whiskey, with a tumbler of hot water, three times a day, with my meals. The only food I take besides meat and eggs is a little boiled rice with cream and molasses, by way of dessert. I have quit walking and running, and travel over the town in a gig. I study scarcely at all, and sleep as much as possible. From these causes I have begun, within three weeks, to feel decidedly better, and I am sanguine in my expectations being able to prosecute my business till the time arise for me to return to the University at Lexington [about 1817], whether I have resolved to go, notwithstanding the death of Dr. Goforth, whether I should get a partner or not. My constitution requires an occasional release from the fatigues of practice, and this cannot be had in any other way so well.

A full diet, exemption from [patient] care and 10 hours sleep in the 24, and no exercise except that of chewing, seems to have had a general and restorative effect on my constitution...my health has been improved very much since we came here. I ascribe it entirely to complete exemption from the fatigues and irregularities of a professional life, and hope by the end of the session, to be prepared for resuming my profession. I already weigh an eighth part more than I did last summer and have not had a paroxysm since I reached Lexington.

Excerpted from a letter [circa 1817] cited in *The Life of Daniel Drake*, by Edward Mansfield. Cincinnati: Applegate & Co., 1855. 123–125.

Reader Reflection

1. *Being self-reflective and scientific, Drake took a broad, multimodal approach to the treatment of his dyspepsia and fatigue of practice: dietary changes, change in activity, ensuring adequate sleep, reducing clinical patient care, and contemplating hiring an associate partner. What does it take for you to live a healthy life? Take a multidimensional approach like Drake: dealing with body, mind, spirit, and social roles.*

5.25 The Calamitous Effects of Intemperance

A fit of drunkenness is a paroxysm of acute disease, which, arising from any other cause would be regarded with dismay. Habitual drinking generates chronic maladies which ultimately extend to all the organs of the body. It inflames the stomach, the liver, and brain; which are, finally, disorganized. It poisons the whole nervous system; disorders the senses, and palsies the muscles. Thus the entire man is at length transformed, from a condition of health and vigor, to a state of loathsome disease; and the grave is, at last, the only purifier.

In the mind, the side effects of intemperance are equally conspicuous. It impairs the power of observation, weakens attention, renders the memory treacherous, excites the imagination, and subverts the understanding. Neither the observations nor the judgments of one in this condition are to be trusted; they may be correct, but are always liable to be false....

The perverting effects of intemperance on the heart are not less than on the head. It transforms equanimity into petulance; aggravates impatience into irascibility; engenders suspicion; blasts the domestic affections; and converts a good husband and father into a capricious and cruel scourge. It generates a taste for dissolute society, with its diversified obscenities; vulgarizes the feelings; inflames every resentment; introduces the language of profanity, and ends, by establishing habits of falsehood and treachery.

An Oration on the Causes, Evils, and Preventives of Intemperance. Columbus: Olmstead & Bailhache, Printers, 1831.

READER REFLECTION

1. *Here Drake describes the impact a disease, such as alcoholism, can have not just on the functioning of many body organs but also on the mind and the social functioning of a person. Knowledge of the ravages of alcohol on the body is not sufficient to prevent or manage the problem. Discuss the individual, community, and social interventions needed to prevent and treat such diseases.*

5.26 BE ABLE TO DESCRIBE THE NATURAL HISTORY OF A DISEASE: MILK SICKNESS

[Milk sickness] attacks men, woman, and children in equal degree; young children are said to be less liable.

When the individual is about to be taken down, he feels weary, trembles more or less under exertion, and often experiences pain, numbness, and slight cramps in the calves and other muscles of the legs. At the same time, he becomes active; and under fatigue, is likely to experience a slight degree of nausea. His appetite is not generally impaired, but he has a feeling of depression and burning, at the pit of the stomach. He is irresolute, and as much indisposed to mental as to bodily effort. He may continue in this situation for a while and recover spontaneously, or by a single cathartic; but more commonly under the influence of an exciting cause, server symptoms supervene. A full meal, or a great quantity of indigestible food is such a one; but another, far more common and efficient, is violent or protracted muscular exertion. This is, indeed, the only exciting cause, which all the people of the district, concur in admitting. The patient being subjected to this, full vomiting supervenes, with much epigastric distress. He throws up the contents of his stomach; and continuing, at short intervals, to vomit or retch, brings up small quantities of acid and mucous, but very seldom much bile. In attempting to sit up, his sickness increases, and his muscles generally become affected with a twitching and tumultuary [haphazard] motion. In lying he is restless, and tosses himself from side to side, in great anxiety. His thirst is generally unquenchable. In the midst of these symptoms his bowels remain torpid, without pain, and do not swell, but seem rather reduced in volume, with a retraction of the umbilicus towards the spine; so that the pulsations of the aorta can be distinctly perceived. Dr. Thomas McGarraugh, now of Franklin, Ross county, but for many years an observing practitioner, of Washington, Fayette county, states, that the tongue is sometimes natural, but at others pale and covered with a film of mucous, which is yellow in the middle; in the advanced stages of certain violent cases it looks like a mass of raw flesh. The heart manifests a convulsive action, and the aorta pulsates with unwonted violence. Notwithstanding all this, the pulse is sometimes almost natural, and although in certain cases increased in tension, it is not apt to be very frequent. Now and then its diameter becomes very small. These are the remarks of Dr. Toland, which in the main, correspond with those of other observers. There is no cough; but the patient sighs, and his breath has a singular offensive, somewhat mercurial odor; so distinct from that of autumnal fever or any other known disease, as to be regarded quite characteristic of this. The skin is generally cool, in the latter stages cold; Dr. McGarraugh has, however, in some cases observed increased heat on the thorax. The surface generally is always dry.

Many cases are cured, when the symptoms here enumerated are present; but others go on to a fatal termination. In such, the irritability of the stomach is often so great, that the least motion in bed, or a moment's conversation, will bring on retching or vomiting; when, in several instances, the patient has thrown up dark colored matter, like that ejected in fatal cases of yellow fever;—death does not, however, so constantly follow this discharge, as it does the coffee ground evacuation in that disease. The constipation continues and the retraction of the umbilicus rather increases than diminishes. There is no peritoneal soreness on pressure; even the epigastrium does not appear to be particularly tender, but pressure upon it is apt to excite vomiting. The sighing becomes deeper, and a hiccough supervenes, which is not always followed by death. The pulse gradually sinks in fullness and force, but the struggling movement of the heart, and the convulsive or throbbing action of the aorta are rather augmented than abated. The visage of the patient, seldom red in the earlier stages, now becomes deathly pale and shrunken. He tosses less, becomes listless, indifferent to what is passing round him, and often lies, between his fits of retching, in a mild coma. Very seldom is there any delirium; he answers well, and does not often mutter when left to himself; there is, however, a peculiar feebleness of attention, inasmuch as many who have recovered from this advanced stage of the disease, and were supposed, at the time, to be cognizant of all that passed around them, were found afterwards not to remember much of what had transpired; not even the death of relatives, who died from the same disease in the same rooms with themselves. We need not follow these symptoms further, as they bring us to the stage when, from the approach of death, the phenomena must be nearly the same, as in the close of all other maladies. The length of time through which the disease runs, to its termination in recovery or death, varies exceedingly in different cases. In some it comes to a favorable termination within twenty-four hours after the vomiting sets in;—again, that with the other symptoms, continues violent for a week or more and then ceases. Death, also, occurs at every period from the second or third day, up to the end of the second week.

[This is the disease that caused the death of Abraham Lincoln's mother, Sarah Hanks Lincoln.]

"A Memoir on the Diseases Called by the People 'Trembles,' and the 'Sick-Stomach' or 'Milk-Sickness'; as They Have Occurred in the Counties of Fayette, Madison, Clark, and Green in the State of Ohio." *Western Journal of Western Journal of Medicine and Surgery* 3 (1841): 176–179.

READER REFLECTION

1. *This selection is an example of studying a medical condition by observation, analyzing and interpreting the data, considering the wider context of information, and then summarizing it for dissemination. This is not just the method of a scientist or physician but also a method to gain understanding in our work and in life. Consider a problem you would like to understand better and try this approach.*

⬚ 5.27 A Case of Depression Beginning with Burn Trauma and Ending with Outdoor Exercise

The Readers of the *Western Journal* will recollect, that in the Autumn of 1828, its publication was suspended, in consequence of a burn which the Editor received on both hands in extricating one of his female relatives from the flames. The object of this paper is to report such facts connected with that casualty, as may be interesting to the profession.

Case 1. A young lady, aged 20 years, in feeble health, was extensively burned, by her mosquito curtains and calico bed cover being set on fire, after she had fallen asleep. The flames enveloped her head, neck, and arms, and were not extinguished for 20 or 30 seconds. Ardent spirits were first applied, then flaxseed oil, and, lastly, a calcareous soap of the same oil and lime water. Laudanum [an opiate] was administered freely, both externally and internally.

The pain and smarting were intense. Great coldness soon came on, with a weak pulse, and epigastric anxiety. Her mental faculties continued unimpaired. In a short time her respiration became irregular, and stertorous [gasping]. Coma supervened; and about 8 hours after the accident she expired. No reaction took place, and she died from shock which her nervous system suffered....

Case 2. The Editor, in rescuing the patient whose case has just been related, was severely burned in both hands. It happened by compressing the burning clothes in his naked hands, until the flames extinguished....

There resulted, however, from this local injury a great constitutional disturbance.... Of course so grave an accident was more likely to be followed by a state of nervous...irritation, and this in its most distressing form, actually supervened. Several causes seem to have conspired to depress the energy and disorder the sensibilities of the nervous system.

1. The acute sensibility of the parts injured, result as in the case of medical men generally, from the use of the hands in a great variety of delicate manipulations. In consequence of this state of exalted sensibility, the pain, for several hours after the accident, was excruciating, notwithstanding the liberal use of laudanum.

2. The scene of the concentrated horror, under which the injury was inflicted, contributed not a little to overthrow the powers of the nervous system.

3. The immersion of both hands, extensively denuded of cuticle, in a liniment of oil and white lead, seems to have contributed largely to the same effect. The direct influence of the preparations of lead on the nerves of the part to which they are applied and through them upon the system at large is unquestionable....

The morbid states of the secretory organs were sufficiently indicative of an overthrow of the functions of that system, which presides over their various operations; but the feelings of the patient were still more significant of nervous depression and perversion. A sense of muscular debility and a consciousness of mental imbecility, extreme restlessness, and morbid vigilance, were the utterable sensations which can be recollected. None of the ordinary stimuli of life, either moral or physical, produced their characteristic effects, the system being insensible to their presence, or the effects which they produced being different from those which they excite in health. In short, every sensation, both of mind and body, was unpleasant if not painful; and this continued to be the case for at least five weeks....

It is, also, worthy of being stated, that for a twelve-month or more after the accident, the cerebral affection was nearly suspended, but has since that time been gradually returning, though it is much less severe than before the burn....

I have been more prolix in these details, because those states of chronic nervous irritation, which no medicine can cure, are common; may spring from various causes, afflict persons of both sexes and of different ages, subject the unfortunate patient to the derision of his acquaintances, and too often bring upon his constitution the desolating tortures of officious [annoying] medication. I have seen many persons in this sad and pitiless state of physical and moral imbecility, and can bear testimony to the great uncertainty of medical prescriptions for their relief; indeed, I have often known them augment the very irritation they are expected to subdue; and am compelled to believe, that many of the nervous diseases which are so often prolonged through an indefinite period, are kept up by our *polypharmacia antispasmodica* [use of multiple antispasmotic drugs].

In these cases, so distressing to the patient and so perplexing to the physician, the best resource is exercise in the open air, with an abandonment of all active and irritating medicines. In many instances the plan will be of difficult execution, for the patient will be alarmed at the very suggestion of exercise; but it soon recommends itself by its very beneficial effects, and if no organ is permanently deranged in structure, it will, by perseverance, work out its cure.

"History of Two Cases of Burn, Producing Serious Constitutional Irritation." *Western Journal of the Medical and Physical Sciences* 4 (1830): 48–60.

READER REFLECTION

1. These case reports are remarkable for the descriptions of his sister-in-law's development of septic shock due to her burn, his development of depression in response to his burns, what it took for him to recover from his depression, and his critique and limitations of current medical approaches. He ended by saying stop the medicines that are not working and exercise in the open air while fully recognizing the patient would likely resist. Sometimes less is more. The challenge is knowing when. Do you have a situation where you have tried all sorts of approaches and see little progress or improvement? Consider pulling back and trying a simpler approach.

❇ 5.28 DESCRIPTION OF POST-TRAUMATIC NEURALGIA FOLLOWING A SEVERE BURN

As the period of cicatrization [process of wound healing to produce scar tissue] approached, the granulations became affected with a distressing neuralgia, which was violent, for six or eight months, and has not yet, at the end of nearly two years, entirely ceased. It would be difficult to characterize the different kinds of pain which the patient endured for the first half of this period. Sometimes it was dull and aching, but oftener acute and suddenly radiated from a point through the whole eschar [dry, dark scab/dead tissue caused by burn]. At other times, it resembled the sensation produced in the extremities of a nerve, by pressure or a blow on its trunk; again, it was a sense of formication [sense of small ants crawling under the skin], and then of urtication [intense itching]; but more commonly the patient could only compare it with the imaginary effect of millions of fine, red hot needles, running in all directions through the new flesh. Its onset was frequently sudden, and almost as transient, as an electric shock; suggesting to the mind of the patient, that it might be owing to the imperfect conducting power of the new nerves. Throughout the whole period, the parts were liable, at times, to a sense of violent spasmodic contraction, and in this condition, if pressed upon, felt almost as hard as cartilage. Several circumstances were observed to exert and influence on this affection.

1. When the patient was dyspeptic or otherwise indisposed, it was apt to be more violent.

2. When the parts were long exposed to the cold, it was made worse. Their calefacient power [sensation of warmth] was, and remains greatly reduced....

3. When the hands were hung down, the neuralgia was suddenly and insupportably aggravated. For several months it appeared to the patient, upon letting

his left hand fall by his side, that its continuance in that position would excite general convulsions—such were his feelings on the subject. If, however, he held a weight, or grasped any solid body, the distress was less poignant.

4. For many months, a kind of neuralgic flash or explosion was the invariable consequence of a deep inspiration, whether made in sneezing, coughing, sighing, or as an experiment. Stuck with this effect, the patient verified it by innumerable observations, and was not long in discovering (what seemed to render the fact still more curious) that the shock produced by a second deep inspiration, was much less, than that attendant on the first; and that upon continuing to respire, in that manner, a third and fourth time, the neuralgia would cease to be reproduced. After a few minutes, however, it could be re-excited by the same means, with its characteristic violence. I state the fact without attempting its explanation.

5. The effect of pressure on this neuralgia was highly beneficial, but relief ceased with compression. It was surprising to the patient, to observe how much compression the recent granulations and eschar could sustain, without any un-pleasant sensation—but the reverse. For months he was under the necessity of devising new modes of applying pressure, as the situation of the parts affected rendered every contrivance imperfect in its operation, and he was often obliged to seize and powerfully compress the principal eschar with the other hand so as to relieve the neuralgia when it became insupportable. For several weeks after cicatrization had commenced, the patient could not sleep at night, without placing the left hand under his pillow, in such a manner that the weight of his head would rest upon the eschar.

"History of Two Cases of Burn, Producing Serious Constitutional Irritation." *Western Journal of the Medical and Physical Sciences* 4 (1830): 48–60.

READER REFLECTION

1. *Here is a highly engaged patient (Drake himself) conducting trial-and-error approaches to find relief from severe, disabling pain. This went on for two years, and many individuals would have become discouraged and stopped. Drake continued and eventually became highly productive once again. What character qualities enable a person to work through such a severe trauma and regain function while others succumb and are never the same?*

✖ 5.29 Nature Therapy

Everywhere on the shores of the lakes, from Ontario to Superior, if the general atmosphere be calm and clear, there is, in summer, a refreshing lake and land breeze; the former commencing in the forenoon, and with the capricious temper, continuing through most of the day; the latter setting in a night, after the radiation from the ground has reduced its heat below that of the water. These breezes are highly acceptable to the voyager a while in the lower Lake region, and by no means to be despised after he reaches the upper.

But the summer climate of the lakes, is not the only source of benefit to invalids; for the agitation imparted by the boat, on voyages of several days duration, through waters which are never stagnant, and sometimes rolling, will be found among the most efficient means of restoring health, in many chronic diseases, especially those of a nervous character, such as hysteria and hypochondriasm.

Another source of benefit is the excitement imparted by the voyage to the faculty of observation. At a watering place all the features of the surrounding scenery are soon familiarized to the eye, which then merely wanders over the comingled throngs of valetudinarians, doctors, dancers, idlers, gamblers, coquettes and dandies, whence it soon returns, to inspect the infirmities or *Tedium vitae* (weariness of life) of its possessor; but on protracted voyages, through new and fresh regions, curiosity is stirred up to the highest pitch, and pleasantly gratified by the hourly unfolding of fresh aspects of nature; some new blending of land and lake—a group of islands different from the last—aquatic fields of wild rice and lilies—rainbow walking on the "face of the deep"—a waterspout, or a shifting series of painted cloud seen in the kaleidoscope of heaven.

The Northern Lakes: A Summer Residence for Invalids of the South. Louisville, KY: J. Maxwell Jr., 1842.

Reader Reflection

1. There is a health benefit of being out in nature and getting away from the stresses of the work life. When was the last time you took a hike or visited a lake and rested? Is it a habit?

✖ 5.30 First Report of the Ohio Lunatic Asylum

Of the Ohio Lunatic Asylum, in Columbus, we know much more having lately received the Annual Report to the Legislature, by its Director and Superintendent.

This is the first report, made after the opening of the Infirmary, and comprises the year from November, 1838 to November, 1839.

During that time, 157 patients were admitted concerning whom we extract the following tabular view.

Patients admitted into the Asylum from 30th November 1838 to 15th November 1839

Males	*87*
Females	*70*

Age when admitted

Under 20 years	*7*
Between 20–30 years	*71*
Between 30–40 years	*41*
Between 40–50 years	*20*
Between 50–60 years	*14*
Between 60–70 years	*2*

Paupers	*125*
Pay patients	*48*

Single	*88*
Married	*56*
Widows	*11*
Widowers	*2*

Type of insanity

Mania	*101*
Melancholic variety	*17*
Epileptic	*12*
Homicidal	*4*
Moral insanity	*0*
Incoherence/Dementia	*10*
Idiotism or Imbecility	*3*

Supposed remote or exciting causes

Intemperance	*7*
Domestic affliction	*6*
Puerperal [post-partum]	*13*

Ill health of various kinds	*14*
Loss of friends	*4*
Matrimonial perplexities	*4*
Fright	*3*
Intense application	*3*
Jealousy	*2*
Disappointed love	*10*
Epilepsy	*9*
Injuries to head	*5*
Constitutional	*10*
Disappointment and mortification	*10*
Masturbation (produced and perpetuated by the practice)	*16*
Fear of want, loss of property, etc.,	*7*
Ill treatment of parents or guardians	*2*
Religious excitement and anxiety, including perplexity, exaltation, enthusiasm, fanaticism, doubt and fear of future punishment.	*15*
Unknown	*7*

Discharges

Recovered	*27*
Incurable	*5*
Idiotic	*2*
Eloped	*1*
Died	*8*
Total	*43*

Prospects of those remaining in the Asylum

Entirely favorable	*15*
Favorable	*15*
Doubtful	*34*
Unfavorable	*50*

The edifice is situated one mile east of Columbus in the midst of ample grounds, and in a healthy locality. It is the most extensive building, we suppose, in the Valley of the Mississippi, and fashioned after the best models of the Eastern States. The whole discipline of the establishment is mild and paternal. All restraint, not absolutely necessary, is avoided, and every moral influence is pressed into the treatment of the unfortunate inmates. The Superintendent, Dr. Awl, has made the management of the Lunatic Asylums a special study, and is unwearied in his efforts, for the comfort and care of all the patients—facts which we do not derive from the Report, so much as from other sources, and especially personal observation. It is proper to state, for the benefit of persons at a distance, that Columbus may be reached, either from the north or south, by the Ohio and Erie Canal, which, as it crosses the State from Cleveland to Portsmouth, is connected with Columbus.

"Lunatic Asylums." *Western Journal of Medicine and Surgery* 1 (1840): 380–384.

READER REFLECTION

This report describes the state of thinking in 1840 about severe mental health problems leading to loss of role and psychological functioning and that resulted in institutionalization. Treatment of severe cases was in a new asylum for the entire state of Ohio, and he was alerting his fellow physicians that the asylum was available.

1. *What is available to treat severe mental health problems in your community? How do we treat mental illness (or not treat them) now? How well resourced? Are there gaps? How could treatment of mental illness be improved?*

5.31 DIAGNOSING AND PREDICTING THE CHOLERA EPIDEMIC

Leaving the Old World, we come to contemplate epidemic Cholera in the New.

From the gazettes, it appears that on 9th of June, of the present year, a malignant *Cholera morbus* suddenly broke out at Quebec, among the Canadian French, and wretched immigrants, chiefly from Ireland, who had, during the spring, been thrown in thousands upon the banks of the St. Lawrence. It quickly spread over the city, and affected many of the natives in comfortable circumstances. In a few days it was at its height, and before two weeks, had sensibly declined; indeed, nearly ceased. On the 11th or 12th, the same malady manifested itself in Montreal, 120 miles further up the St. Lawrence, where it raged with great mortality; but on 24th of June was nearly extinct. Meantime it made its appearance in many of the villages surrounding these two cities; and affected the Canadian French still more, it is said, than immigrants, multitudes of whom had ascended the river as far as Montreal, and even above.

The question has been started, whether this be anything else, than the ordinary endemic of the country, in an aggravated form? It is impossible, from the data, which have, as yet, reached Cincinnati, to resolve this question; From the suddenness of the invasion, and its short duration, the multitudes taken down, its great prevalence among the poor and exposed, its alarming mortality, and the concourse of symptoms, I am compelled, until other facts shall be made public, to regard it as an extension of the Asiatic epidemic. The question whether it will extend into the United States, from Canada, will probably be answered in the affirmative, before these pages see the light. For whether propagated by contagion or atmospheric influence of any kind, its entrance into our country is not likely to be prevented, unless the laws of its diffusion should be different in America from those of Europe and Asia.

A Practical Treatise on the History, Prevention, and Treatment of Epidemic Cholera, Designed Both for the Profession and the People. Cincinnati: Cory and Fairbank, 1832. 23, 24.

READER REFLECTION
What Drake did here was gather as much primary data as he could about the cholera epidemic from Asia and Europe and track its movement into Canada before it ever reached the United States. It arrived in Cincinnati less then ninety days after Drake published this treatise. This is an excellent example of staying abreast of what was happening in other parts of the world that would impact the local community and seeking to be proactive about it. Influenza, another epidemic disease, is monitored this way every year with new vaccines against specific types of influenza created and used.
1. *What is happening in other parts of the world right now that can impact your work and your community—either positively or negatively?*

✖ 5.32 ANALYZING DATA TO REACH A VALID CONCLUSION
Poisonous air [miasma, pollution], formed by the decomposition of dead vegetable and animal matters, acted on by heat and moisture, has with confidence been cited as the remote cause [of cholera]. In support of this theory, it has been alleged and with truth, that the disease prevails most in hot and humid situations, which are supposed to send forth miasmatic exhalations; in close, dirty, and ill ventilated cities; that the season of the year when intermittent and remittent fevers, said to depend

on malaria, are prevalent. It has, moreover, not infrequently put on, after the first paroxysms and, the type of one of them, or some other fever. Thus, the miasmatic theory is far more comfortable to the ascertained fact, than either of the others just mentioned, and deserves grave consideration. When we recollect, however, that in several instances it has prevailed in dry places and at great elevations; it has continued, in some cases, throughout the winter; that it is, and always has been, absent from many places on the surface of the globe, where heat, moisture, and decomposable matter, all the necessary requisites for the generation of [poisonous air], abound, I am unable to ascent to the miasmatic hypothesis although so plausibly supported.

A Practical Treatise on the History, Prevention, and Treatment of Epidemic Cholera, Designed Both for the Profession and the People. Cincinnati: Cory and Fairbank, 1832. 27.

READER REFLECTION

1. *Frequently we need to draw a conclusion based on limited or incomplete information. To arrive at what is most plausible requires thinking systematically with the information we have to draw inferences. This is a higher order processing of data. Consider a situation you have faced or are facing where you had/have limited information but need to draw a conclusion. What mental process of critical analysis will you use to help you reach the most plausible conclusion that best fits the data?*

2. *This sort of hypothesis generation and clinical reasoning with data is what physicians do many times every day. How does a person become proficient with clinical reasoning?*

✖ 5.33 FACTORS IN THE PATIENT'S PREDISPOSITION SHAPE THE "HOST RESPONSE"

Let us turn from the fruitless pursuit of a principal and universal remote cause of epidemic Cholera, to the more profitable study of auxiliary causes. These, in theory, may be referred to two divisions; first, such as favor the generation or exalt the activity of the specific remote cause; and secondly, such as predispose the body to its action, or quicken it into life. Every auxiliary cause must act in one of these two modes; but, after having established the classes, it may be difficult to assort the agents, which are to be distributed....

The circumstances which predispose the body to the action of that agent, whatever it may be, and are, exhaustion from age, chronic infirmities, and un-nutritious diet; intemperance in the use of ardent spirits; long-continued exertion; confined lodgings; the habitual breathing of impure air; exposure to the damp and cool atmosphere of the night, after intense heat of the day; irregular and excessive indulgence in food; apprehension of the disease; grief from the loss of friends; finally, constitutional temperament or native predisposition. The influence of these circumstances is so great, that those who are under several, or even one of them, are in great danger of being seized when the disease prevails; but it may occur in persons who are exempt from the operation of the whole, except the last, and there is, therefore, a cause distinct from them all, and their agency is limited to the effect of predisposing the system to its action.

A Practical Treatise on the History, Prevention, and Treatment of Epidemic Cholera, Designed Both for the Profession and the People. Cincinnati: Cory and Fairbank, 1832. 49, 50.

Reader Reflection

1. *Through observation Drake drew the conclusions that a) not all people exposed to a disease producing agent get sick from it, and b) that each individual has predisposing factors that will influence whether they get sick or not. Note the factors that he has identified and how they are still relevant today. Are there others?*

2. *How is it that grief from the loss of friends or family predisposes an individual to become ill? Discuss how to respond to such a loss that makes it less likely for a person to become ill.*

5.34 The Three-Year Experience of Cholera in Cincinnati and Lessons Learned This Far

The whole number of deaths in Cincinnati, for six months beginning with April, in the years 1831, '32, '33, will appear from the following table:

	1831	1832	1833
April	55	77	0
May	45	110	107
June	92	95	154
July	102	116	373
August	128	141	177
September	93	97	95
Total	515	636	956

If we deduct from the mortality of the present year the Cholera returns, we have a remainder of 586, which is little more than the mean term of the two preceding years.

Among the complications with Cholera this summer, the most important was dysentery. The number of cases has been considerable, though the deaths for six months were only 13. In some instances the disease commenced as Cholera, and terminated in dysentery—in others the reverse; while a few exhibited many of the characteristic symptoms of both, at the same time. In proportion as the dysenteric character predominated, was the safety of the patient. The treatment which this dysentery required was substantially the same with that of Cholera. Calomel and opium combined were the indispensable parts of the *methodus medendi* [description and treatment of diseases]; but mucillages—oleo-saccharums—cretaceous mixtures, and different preparations of rhubarb, were valuable auxiliaries. In some cases, astringents were of service.

In conclusion, I shall repeat for the hundredth time, that all who would be cured of Epidemic Cholera should commence the treatment in its first and diarrheal stage. Almost any method, provided rest be a part, will then succeed; while no means yet discovered can be relied on, after vomiting and spasms have supervened; and this is all that is of any substantial practical value, in the thousand and odd volumes which have been written on this malady. Such at least is my opinion.

"Epidemic Cholera." *Western Journal of Medicine and Surgery* 7 (1833): 161–181.

READER REFLECTION

1. *The summary of deaths due to cholera in this three-year period represents about 5–8 percent of the population in Cincinnati. What are the common causes of death in your community? What is being done to intervene and reduce the deaths due to these conditions?*

5.35 THOUGHTS ON HOW MEDICINES WORK AND OPIUM AS A SELECTED EXAMPLE

Few subjects in the profession involve greater difficulties than the *Modus Operandi* of Medicines. The effects of almost every medicine are various—the mode of its operation complex and obscure. Were the human body a single molecule, homogeneous in structure and function, the laws of its relations with surrounding objects would be few and easily comprehended. But the reverse of this is true, and hence the inevitable failure of all who have sought to embrace, in a few general propositions, the principles which relate to the subject.

It must be granted that some of these propositions are, on the whole, correct; as, for instance, that which pronounces all medicines to be *alterants*; but this merely declares them active substances in relation to our systems; and leaves us ignorant of the variety of alterations which they can produce, and of the modes of that production, although these are the proper objects of inquiry. As the organs which compose the body have different aptitudes and are variously acted on by the same agent, we shall find that the medicine which excites one function, may disturb another, suspend a third, and leave a fourth unaffected—and as organs are associated and cooperative, if one [organ] is changed in its actions, others will likewise experience change,—finally, every substance in nature exerting upon us an action peculiar to itself, the changes, both primary and secondary, which are wrought out by medicinal agents are exceedingly numerous. I shall proceed to consider in what way they are brought about.

This inquiry naturally divides itself into two parts:

1. How is it that a medicine applied directly to an organ changes its mode of existence?

2. In what manner does this change cause an alteration in the mode of existence of other organs?

With respect to the first, we can only say, that the effects of an external agent upon the functions of an organ, provided it acts neither mechanically nor chemically, are referable to the existence, in the organ, of the properties denominated sensibility and contractility, without one or both of which no phenomenon would follow its application. Beyond this, I presume our analysis of the subject cannot be carried. A knowledge of *quomodo* [how] is evidently unattainable. We can only observe and register the feelings and symptoms which follow the contact of the medicine....

[A] mode in which medicines produce an effect in parts remote from that to which we apply them, is by being absorbed into the sanguiferous system, circulated with the blood, and finally eliminated, through the excretory organs.... But what the living body will or will not tolerate, we can only know from experiment and observation; and by these we learn, that active substances thrown upon the mucous membranes, and, under certain circumstances, upon the skin, are absorbed, do circulate, cause disturbance of the functions, and are finally eliminated through some of the excretory outlets of the sanguiferous system.... It is not my design to exhibit a catalogue of substances which, taken into the stomach, have been detected in the blood, or in the secreted fluids of the kidneys, lungs, or skin. More then twenty may be enumerated, without referring to writers of a period, when experiments in physiology were conducted less rigidly than at the present time. Indeed, facts of this kind have become numerous, and are so authentic, that no one can venture to deny them....

The mode of action and effects of opium are still more complex and diversified. When take in a large but not deleterious portion, the following are its characteristic effects:

1. The excitement of the system at large, is exalted;—the contractions of the heart are rendered more frequent and vigorous, the cerebral functions more animated.

2. Drowsiness presently supervenes, the organs of sense become obtuse, the functions of the brain are reduced in energy, the actions of the heart are rendered slow and deliberate, with a soft and full pulse.

3. Slight diaphoresis [sweating], with itching, terminates the series of effects.

Here we have many successive constitutional disturbances, and they afford prima facie evidence of a complicated modus operandi. There is, I think, a little to require or sustain the belief, that they all spring immediately from the impress of opium on the mucous membranes of the stomach. That the first are referable, directly and indirectly, to such impress, is extremely probable; but the second, it appears to me, arise from the transmission of the medicine to the heart and brain, and other internal organs; the last from its elimination through the skin.

Thus, the medicine acts on the stomach as an excitant, and by correspondence of function, propagates to its effects on the brain and heart. They being excited, transmit to the organs over which they preside, and reciprocally to each other, an increased quantity of their respective influences, and hence, by dependence of function, more exalted vital properties and a higher grade of excitement, manifest themselves in the system generally. At length the medicine is absorbed, and enabled to act directly upon the brain and heart, when the sensibility and contractility of these and the other organs, are diminished, and the second class of effects which I have enumerated, ensue. Finally, it is thrown out of the system, through the skin, and some disturbance of feeling and function in that organ, is the consequence of its presence.

[*Materia medica* was the term used in Drake's time to describe knowledge about the therapeutic properties of substances used in medical practice prior to pharmacology. This selection was written six years after the first College of Pharmacy was created in 1821 in Philadelphia and twenty-three years before a College of Pharmacy was established in Cincinnati (1850).]

"Observations and the Modus Operandi and Effects of Medicines." *Western Journal of the Medical and Physical Sciences* 1 (1827): 249–263.

READER REFLECTION

1. *Opium had been used for thousands of years and in Drake's lifetime would be a cause of the Opium War (1839–1842) between China and Britain and continues to cause problems for society. How big a problem is opium's derivatives (heroin and prescription narcotics) in your community? What is being done about this problem?*

5.36 PUBLIC HEALTH WHILE TRAVELING ON THE RIVERS: THREE RECOMMENDATIONS

Steamboat Bars. Now, that ardent spirits are no more seen on the dinner tables of our steamers, and the number of passengers, who desire or dare to frequent the bars, is greatly reduced, it would seem to be natural, and not difficult, to suppress them entirely. The chief motive for retaining them is destroyed, when they yield but little profit, and, therefore, the owners of the boats might be expected not to resist their abolition. But under what influence can this important reform be brought about? We answer, that of the friends of temperance, exerted on the general government. After having legislated on the registration and inspection of steamboats, even to a prescription for tiller chains, it would be no unwarrantable exercise of power to suppress the sale of intoxicating drinks, both to passengers and operatives. The principle on which Congress might place this interposition, is the same as that on which they have directed chains for ropes—the safety of passengers. No observing man can believe but that man of the disasters which have happened to our steamboats were the effect of intemperance, particularly indulged in at night; and that, with its suppression, the number of accidents would be signally abated. We cannot but ardently desire to see the friends of temperance move in this manner.

India Rubber Life-Preservers. On our present voyage down the Ohio and Mississippi, not less than before, we have marveled to see so few of these valuable articles. Hundreds now travel on steamers without them, would, if they had never been invented, deplore the want which they now neglect to supply. With a good life preserver around her chest, even the most helpless and timid woman would be safer for several hours unless the water might chance to be as, it now is, but two or three degrees above the freezing point; and still but few ladies are provided them, and still fewer gentlemen, although none of the former and not many of the latter know how to swim. By the way, it is a serious and absurd defect, in the physical education of our daughters, that they are not taught how to swim; as it is a valuable exercise early in life, and a source of confidence and security even to old age. In past times, when our women remained at home, because they could not travel, the latter consideration was of less moment than at present, when so many perform long voyages, at every moment exposed to casualties which might drown them, merely because a day had not been devoted to their instruction in the art of swimming.

Steamboat Explosions. All passengers who are exposed to these accidents ought to know, that the steam which spreads through the cabin, when explosions occur, will not scald those parts of the body which are covered even thinly. Thus, those, who are in their berths when such an accident happens, should lie still, and cover up their heads, instead of rising, as so often happened; and those who are up, might protect themselves by covering their hands and face with an apron, the skirts of a coat, or even a silk handkerchief. Reaching the skin through such fabric, steam, which would otherwise blister, will scarcely redden it. A further precaution, not unworthy of notice, is to suspect or hold the breath, at the moment of becoming enveloped in the steam, by which its introduction into the larynx and lungs is prevented.

"Traveling Editorial." *Western Journal of the Medical and Physical Sciences 7 (1843): 239–240.*

READER REFLECTION

1. *What are the important public health issues of your community needing attention? What practical advice could be offered? Or specific regulations considered to improve public safety?*

✄ 5.37 AN ADVOCATE FOR VACCINATION

The neglect of vaccination, in Ohio, especially by the poorer classes of people, is, or ought to be most alarming. Might not our legislature terminate this cruel apathy? We think they might; and hope they will, for at no distant day, we are likely to have the natural Small Pox superadded to the Epidemic Cholera. Our plan is, that a law should be passed, excluding every child from the benefits of our admirable system of free schools who had not been vaccinated. To prevent complaints, it should not take effect, till six months after its passage, which would afford ample time to have all the children of the state vaccinated; and, those who are very poor, for whom the schools were, indeed, chiefly designed, might not be excluded, it should be made the duty of the overseers of the poor, on the application of parents who have not the means of paying for the operation, to have it done at public expense.

The immediate impulse and permanent stimulus, which this regulation would impart to the practice of vaccination, would, we doubt not, render it universal over the state; and we respectfully commend it to the consideration of newspaper editors, politicians (meaning statesman), and the benevolent of all sects and parties.

"Neglect of Vaccination—Free Schools." *Western Journal of the Medical and Physical Sciences* 7 (1833): 156.

READER REFLECTION

1. *Discussions regarding the pros and cons of vaccination are not new. What are the controversies about vaccinations today?*
2. *What role should the state have in regulating and overseeing the practice of vaccination to prevent disease?*

✶ 5.38 CAUSES OF PROFESSIONAL QUARRELS

The members of every vocation have their peculiar relations, from the proper maintenance of which, results much of their happiness, as well as the dignity and influence, of the body which they compose. The causes which disturb the harmony of those, who, in the same place, are engaged in a common pursuit, must, of course, vary according to the nature of the pursuit, and are far more operative in some callings than others....

I propose to lay open some of the causes, which generate differences and discord in the [medical] profession, as I have either observed or felt their operation.

1. Rivalship is a predisposing cause, (and sometimes the only one) of much collision among physicians and surgeons....

2. Envy, a passion which prevails in all ranks of society, is not less operative in the medical profession, than elsewhere; and originates not a few of the personal disputes which agitate it....

3. Differences of opinion, on the principles of the profession, lead to many of the personal antipathies and controversies which disturb the profession; and, to a greater or lesser extent, involve the feelings of society.

4. The establishment of medical schools is a prolific source of discord in the profession.... [T]here are at the present time, nearly a hundred medical professors in the United States, and at least a thousand physicians, who in their own and the opinion of their friends, are as well, or better qualified, to fill professional chairs. These two great classes, of course, stand in relation to each other, which predisposes them to hostility.

5. The people themselves occasion not a few jealousies and strifes of medical men. Almost every family has its physician, who is generally pronounced more skillful, or courteous, or attentive, than the man in whom the neighbor confides. This comparative praise seldom fails to reach the ear of him who is thus depreciated; and, by a natural association of ideas, he connects the idol of the family with the idolators; and comes to dislike the person, whom he thinks unjustly elevated at his expense. But still worse, the enthusiast admirers of a particular physician will often collect and circulate petty scandal, and sometimes actual falsehoods, on a rival of their favorite; to which he will give the countenance which results from silence, when he should, in fact, be the first to step forth in the defense of him, who is thus assailed. Professional fame is the capital of a physician, and he must not suffer it to be purloined even should its defense involve him quarrels.

6. As neighboring physicians practice indiscriminately, throughout the same community, many occasions for misunderstanding or actual hostility, will necessarily arise. They are in perpetual competition, and every thing which maintains the contests is personal; its immediate object is public favor, its remote, the acquisition of property.

7. Undercharging is a source of personal difficulty among physicians....

8. Quackery of other kinds not infrequently disturbs the repose of the profession. Its members are so numerous, that among them there must always be some, who are willing to recommend themselves, by the arts of *charlatanerie*; the influence of which on many persons is irresistible. It is the duty of the honorable members of the profession, to expose and condemn such impostures. But this is never done, without exciting strike and turmoil....

9. When a physician is sick or absent, another is of necessity called in by his patients, if they need advice. This sometimes leads to open animosities. He who is summoned to this vicarious function may aim at retaining himself permanently in the place of the other....

10. Consultations are copious sources of personal difficulty in the profession. Great reliance is, generally placed by the patient, or his friends, on the consulting physician, because the other is presumed to have exhausted his skill.... The consulting physician, moreover, is often questioned, apart from the other, on the past treatment and the probable issue of the case; when, if deficient in honor, he is apt to say, or look or insinuate, such things as he knows will operate to the injury of his colleague; who of course resents the insidious attack on his character should he discover it....

On the whole, it is not proper for physicians to be enemies of each other; but being such, it is still more improper for them to undertake, conjointly, that which personal enmity can scarcely fail to render unavailing, if not prejudicial to human life.

"Professional Quarrels." In *Practical Essays on Medical Education and the Medical Profession in the United States.* Cincinnati: Roff & Young, 1832. 96–104.

READER REFLECTION

1. Professional quarrels occur in many fields. Are the causes of such quarrels that Drake offers similar in other fields? In your field?

2. Have you experienced a professional "quarrel"? How did you resolve it?

3. Discuss: Who suffers when professional quarrels occur? The individuals? The profession?

5.39 THE COMPENSATION OF PHYSICIANS

The honest earnings of medical men exceed, to an incredible degree, their actual receipts; because they are never without patients of whom they cannot demand any thing. But whence arises the claim of pauperism on the medical profession? We can perceive no obligation resting on the physician to give his services, gratuitously, to a poor family, that is not binding on all who surround such a family, to supply it with the necessaries and comforts of life. The judgment of society on this point is arbitrary and selfish....

The practice of attending the poor gratuitously, and those in moderate circumstances for a slender and uncertain, occasional, compensation, is, however, universal, and not likely to cease. Such being the case, it follows, that the support of a physician must be derived from those who are in comfortable or opulent circumstances; and having made the amount of property an element in the system of charging we should carry it out. If, according to public opinion, the patient who has not the means of paying much, should be charged but little, it follows, that the patient who is wealthy should be charged a great deal. The rule should work both ways. It does not, however, work upward without resistance. The rich man say— you should attend the poor gratuitously, but you must charge me no more than the mechanic who administers to my artificial wants! Admirable consistency!—The impudent offspring of a cold-hearted selfishness. There are three strata in society, the rich, the poor, and the intermediate, which graduate each other. The charges of a physician should be framed with reference to the last. As he descends among the poor, they must decrease till they vanish; as he ascends to the rich, they should be increased, in proportion to their reduction in the other direction. This is just, because it is but carrying out the conventional idea, that poverty should modify our charges. It assumes that if poverty should reduce—riches should augment them— an assumption which cannot be overthrown. We ought to look to our rights in this matter. In every town it should be the practice of physicians, to charge higher as their patients are wealthier; and they should sustain each other in the collection of their claims, on this principle....

Dim, indeed, is the eye of the common sense, in any people, when it cannot perceive, that the physician should be familiarly acquainted with several sciences, all of which, except anatomy and chemistry, are imperfect and speculative; and that, in his practical duties, he is to apply half-formed rules deduced from these sciences, to the abatement of disease, and the restoration of health—duties which require patient observation, sound judgment, and deep penetration. For these he is properly developed, a long and laborious course of study is indispensable, and the taste and temperament of the individual must be molded in a specific manner. His vocation is therefore compatible with any other pursuit. Still further, the physician should be, at all times, intellectually and physically prepared to execute whatever service may be suddenly thrown upon him. How then can he, in justice, to the community, abstract his thoughts from his professional duties, and direct them on any other business? As easily might he serve both God and mammon—as soon direct the movements of the ship in battle, and at the same time amputate the limbs of the wounded.

The genius of the medical profession, excludes then, all other callings, as means of support; it claims the practitioner, both soul and body, as its own; commands him not to wander into the paths of commerce, the mechanic arts or pecuniary speculation; and tells his own conscience and the community, of he should, that he lives in the violation of duty. At the same time, no other profession involves it members in such extensive and varied social relations. In every part of the United States, the physician is, ought to be, a person of high relative rank—he should be a man of letters and science—a gentleman in habits and manners. He cannot, therefore, live in retirement and poverty. Like an actor while the play is advancing, he must be ready at any moment to enter the stage, and is obliged to appear in costume appropriate to his character.

From these premises it results, that the compensation of the physician should be liberal. It ought to bring back with interest what had been expended in the acquisition of elementary knowledge, and afford compensation for the tedious years of probation, to which he was subjected; it should enable him to procure all the necessary books, apparatus, and instruments; provide adequately for the support and education of his family; and secure him against want in his old age.

"Compensation of Physicians." *Western Journal of the Medical and Physical Sciences* 12 (1838): 49–56.

READER REFLECTION

1. *Here is an argument for the use of a sliding scale for paying for services based on the patient's ability to pay. What has happened to that system of payment? Discuss whether this is a just way or not for the patient.*
2. *Should physicians volunteer their services to care for the poor? Why or why not?*

✠ 5.40 IMPROVE UPON YOUR WORK FOR FUTURE GENERATIONS

The causes of failure generally lie in our own weaknesses, of which the greatest is the want of unfaltering constancy. Holding on to the end in any laudable enterprise, is with few exceptions to achieve a triumph. I hope and feel, and believe, that we *shall* steadily hold on, and thus, when some young student, now sitting thoughtful and silent in our midst, shall with age and tottering footsteps, follow the mortal remains of the last of us to the grave, he will say to the physicians of another generation, then assembled around: "Carry forward the noble work which they began, make it better than you found it, and then hand it on to posterity."

"On the Origin and Influences of Medical Periodical Literature and the Benefits of Public Medical Libraries" In *Discourses Delivered by Appointment before the Cincinnati Medical Library Association*. Cincinnati: Moore and Anderson, 1852. 93.

READER REFLECTION

1. *Consider a time when you struggled with persevering through a difficult task, but you persisted and it made all the difference. What enabled you to persevere?*
2. *What work can you improve upon for future generations?*

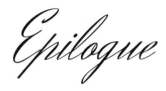

◆ DRAKE'S LEGACY TODAY

How would Daniel Drake's legacy apply to our times? Before answering this question, let's review some of his capacities and his motivation in five human dimensions identified in this book.

Daniel Drake had three foundational capacities that allowed him to understand his world: the ability 1) to *observe*, seeing what is happening around him and identifying social and environmental trends; 2) to *analyze* data based on comparative knowledge; and 3) to rightly *interpret* from his observations and analysis. Drake was a keen observer from his youth, learning to see and explore the natural world of plants and animals through the seasons. He developed a broad knowledge of humanity, his community, and specifically the people who lived there. But he also gained knowledge of what could be by reading widely and visiting other cities and communities. Finally, like a naturalist he interpreted the data he gathered to create a plan of what could be done. Such capacities of observation, analysis, and interpretation remain fundamental and relevant today. Understanding of trends and identifying the needs of our organizations, our neighborhoods, and our communities are necessary to be able to come up with effective approaches to address those needs.

But observing, analyzing, and interpreting is not enough. Drake was *civic-minded*. He was motivated to serve others in order to make their lives better. He did not use his position to take advantage of others for personal gain. He looked for opportunities to create, grow, and improve his community culture. He recognized that becoming involved in building and nurturing institutions and advocating for causes that would benefit society was a good use of his time and talents and, in turn, satisfied a deep-seated motivation. His legacy grew out of this civic spirit as a secondary consequence, not as the primary goal.

Returning to our original question: armed with these capacities and motivation how would Drake's legacy apply in our times? But to set the stage for this inquiry we need to ask, What is happening in our times? What are the major social trends and community needs of this generation?

Most recognize we live in a global, digital age very different from Drake's time, but what is not as obvious is that we are also living in an age of abundance unimaginable in the nineteenth century. Consider the following: Information technology envelops our lives. Knowledge grows at an exponential rate. The standard of living continues to advance with the ubiquity and diffusion of agricultural, manufacturing, and scientific technology. We are surrounded by reams of data, and personal privacy is largely gone. We have ample and varied food. Both prescription and illicit drugs are widely available. We have more guns and more sophisticated and powerful weapons than ever before. Options for entertainment are numerous. The pursuit of leisure and seeking after pleasure is the norm. Legal regulations and rules governing society continue to multiply. We consume more and, in turn, create more waste with increasing impact on the environment. In the midst of all this abundance, the fabric of tightknit communities is more frayed, and even though advances have been made to celebrate diversity and achieve inclusion, community trust is low.

Technology and abundance create challenges. In and of themselves they are neither good nor bad, but they are not morally neutral when we explore the possible consequences. Speaking to a group of computer programmers and scientists in 1992, the late Neil Postman, a professor at New York University, said that "Technology giveth and Technology taketh away. A new technology sometimes creates more than it destroys. Sometimes, it destroys more than it creates. But it is never one-sided." There are always trade-offs. Abundance also brings trade-offs. Abundance creates ease and greater opportunities but also brings more to manage and more decisions on what to do with our time and resources. Our decisions test our character. Society is struggling with the abundance accompanying the digital age.

Consider if Drake were alive today how he might address the following grave issues stemming from abundance and the widespread diffusion of information technology. Though these were not problems of Drake's time, using some of the insights from Drake's example, think about workable solutions. Consider the trade-offs for each of the issues below—what are the positive and negative consequences?

1. *Time management.* Use of information technology devices, for example, smartphones, are ubiquitous. Social media (Instagram, Facebook, Twitter) increasingly captures more and more of our time and attention. The pursuit of

entertainment and virtual, instead of actual, experience and engagement with the world is the norm for many. Managing time in the digital age is increasingly a challenge, robbing attention from other facets of life. The prime technological contributor to physician burnout is the introduction of the electronic health record into medicine, which creates seventy-five minutes more work for every four-hour session of patient care. How can we become more effective at managing our time?

(*Some hints from Drake.* Drake practiced self-discipline and moderation. He was not idle, and he did not engage in activities that wasted his time. He was an early riser and followed a strict schedule, particularly during the academic year. His time was spent on projects and activities that restored him. He did enjoy entertaining guests in his home and remained close to his adult children and grandchildren.)

2. *Picking out useful knowledge in the midst of information noise.* Knowledge grows at an exponential rate, but application of knowledge lags. Some information is misleading or not true. How can we recognize what information is useful and accurate? How can we be critical consumers of information? How can we find information sources?

(*Some hints from Drake.* As a journal editor Drake read widely and sought useful information to pass along to his peers. He had a discerning, critical eye and was not afraid to call out quackery, through his own writings or speeches.)

3. *Managing personal privacy and reputation.* We are surrounded by reams of data and personal privacy is largely gone. How can we use data to help society but at the same time protect individual privacy?

(*Some hints from Drake.* Drake was a person of good character and reputation. He realized his reputation needed to be protected, and he defended it aggressively when his character was unfairly attacked by jealous competitors. Throughout his life he collected data that could be used to improve lives and taught, wrote, and published the knowledge he gained by study and observation.)

4. *Disparities in the midst of plenty.* The standard of living continues to advance with the average income increasing around the world, yet this has not reached all people. Neighborhoods within the same city have wide differences in longevity; in some instances people in one neighborhood live twenty years longer than people from another. How can we address the social and health disparities?

(*Some hints from Drake.* Drake sought to care for the disabled and vulnerable people in his community. His motivation in creating a teaching hospital was out of the need to care for transient individuals who were passing through Cincinnati.)

5. *Addressing public health challenges related to abundance.* Obesity and chronic disease: We have ample food, but not all of it is healthy. The prevalence of obesity and its corresponding adverse effects on health continue to rise. How can we address the obesity epidemic?

The opioid epidemic: Both prescription and illicit drugs are widely available. prescription drugs may be overprescribed; drug addiction is rampant; and the number of deaths due to overdoses is at epidemic levels. How can we address the misuse of drugs and addiction?

Mass shootings: We have more guns and more sophisticated and powerful weapons than ever before. How can we prevent mass shootings?

(*Some hints from Drake.* Drake sought to understand first the contributing causes to public health problems [e.g., cholera, maritime safety, alcoholism]. He realized that these issues were complex and required multilevel interventions including using innovative technologies, drawing on sound science, educating the public, and working with regulatory agencies.)

6. *Seeking to avoid or prevent the adverse impact of consumption on climate and the environment.* We consume more and in turn create more waste. Increased production of greenhouse gases has led to climate change and its adverse impact on the environment and human health. We have mounds of landfills full of items that could last a millennium. How can we be good stewards of the environment?

(*Some hints from Drake.* Drake, the naturalist, appreciated the need to care for and manage the environment and advocated conservancy practices.)

7. *Seeking to build cohesive, trusting communities.* The fabric of tightknit communities is frayed and even though advances have been made to celebrate diversity and achieve inclusion, community trust is low. How can we build cohesive, trusting communities?

(*Some hints from Drake.* Drake was a builder of community culture and focused on institutions, social gatherings, and education as the cornerstones of democratic society. But Drake was a victim of his times in thinking about race—like many in this time period he wrongly believed white people were superior to all other races. At the same time he recognized that love was the great transforming force for humankind to live in harmony, and love was what was needed—learning to love your neighbor as yourself.)

Daniel Drake, because of the legacy that grew out of his life and thought, is a person for all times. Generations come and go, but the lessons of his life continue to endure and are beneficial to all of us.

Daniel Drake

Chronology

October 20, 1785–November 5, 1852

⊠ Becoming a Lifelong Student and Beginning a Medical Career

1785   *October 20. Born in Plainfield, New Jersey, to Isaac Drake and Elizabeth Shotwell Drake, their second child.*

1788   *Age three. Family moves to Mayslick, Kentucky, near the Ohio River. Father farms the land, and Drake sporadically attends school during the winters through age fifteen. He develops a deep appreciation for nature and the outdoors.*

1799   *Age fourteen. In December Drake fulfills the longtime wishes of his father and leaves behind his parents and five siblings—Lizzy age thirteen, Lydia ten, Benjamin six, Lavinia three, and Livingston one—to travel to Cincinnati to study medicine.*

1800   *Age fifteen. Apprenticed for four years to Dr. Goforth of Cincinnati.*

1801   *Age sixteen. Dr. Goforth is the first to introduce cowpox vaccination to prevent small-pox, and Drake was one of his first patients to receive it.*

1802   *Age seventeen. Dr. John Stites joins Dr. Goforth and becomes one of Drake's preceptors. Stites had studied in Philadelphia under Dr. Charles Caldwell and Dr. Benjamin Rush and introduces their discourses and the "young medical science" to Drake.*

1804   *On May 18, at age nineteen, Drake becomes a full partner in the practice of medicine with Dr. Goforth.*

THE FIRST TEN YEARS OF DRAKE'S CLINICAL PRACTICE

1805–1806 *Age twenty. Travels to Philadelphia to study medicine at the University of Pennsylvania (November through March); attends lectures but does not stay through second term for graduation. Lecturers include Drs. Benjamin Rush, Caspar Wistar, Philip Physick, Benjamin Barton, and William Shippen. Drake is exposed to Philadelphia's rich cultural resources.*

1806 *Age twenty-one. Begins practice in Mayslick, Kentucky.*

1807 *Age twenty-two. Returns to Cincinnati to take over Dr. Goforth's practice on April 10. (Goforth had moved to Louisiana.) Marries Harriet Sisson (December 20), niece of Colonel Jared Mansfield (surveyor-general of the Northwest Territory). Founds the Cincinnati Lyceum (a debating society).*

1808 *Age twenty-three. Daughter Harriet is born October 24.*

1809 *Age twenty-four. Daughter Harriet dies September 20, aged eleven months. Drake serves as chairman of the circulating library project committee for Cincinnati.*

1810 *Age twenty-five. On May 2, "Daniel Drake & Co." established in partnership with Drake's brother Benjamin to sell drugs and surgical instruments, groceries, paints, stationary, and books. Publishes* Notices Concerning Cincinnati *May–June, which was an examination of Cincinnati's diseases in context of the environment.*

1811 *Age twenty-six. Son Charles Daniel born April 11. Drake begins building a three-story brick home at 429 East Third Street, Cincinnati.*

1812 *Age twenty-seven. Organizes the First District Medical Society in Cincinnati. Moves into 429 East Third Street, Cincinnati; his home through 1823.*

1813 *Age twenty-eight. Son John Mansfield born. Helps organize the Cincinnati School of Literature and Arts in October.*

1814 *Age twenty-nine. Assists with organizing the Cincinnati Lancaster Seminary. He is the first president of the Circulating Library of Cincinnati the year it opens.*

1815   *Age thirty.* Publishes Natural and Statistical View; or, Picture of Cincinnati and the Miami Country, *which describes the fertile resources of the region with the aim of promoting future settlement and development of Cincinnati and the surrounding region. Sells Daniel Drake & Co. in October, and returns to the University of Pennsylvania to complete his medical degree, attending classes November to March 1816.*

1816   *Age thirty-one. February 5 son John dies age 2¾ years. Receives his medical degree May 16, 1816, from the University of Pennsylvania by special investiture by the Board of Trustees as Drake had missed the final exams. His section on "Medicine" in* Picture of Cincinnati *fulfills his MD thesis requirement. Resumes practice in June 1816 in Cincinnati.*

⊠ BEGINNING AN ACADEMIC CAREER

1817   *Age thirty-two. January 7, accepts the chair of Materia Medica in the medical department of Transylvania University in Lexington, Kentucky. He lasts one term due to conflicts with teaching colleagues and a desire to return to Cincinnati; resigns March 24. Daughter Elizabeth Mansfield is born May 31. Dr. Coleman Rogers joins his practice in Cincinnati July 9; Drake and Rogers announce they will accept medical students for apprenticeship.*

1818   *Age thirty-three. Elected to the American Philosophical Society and the American Antiquarian Society.*

1819   *Age thirty-four. January 19, Drake secures approval by the Ohio General Assembly for charters for a Medical College of Ohio and for a Cincinnati College empowered to grant degrees (the beginning of the University of Cincinnati). Birth of daughter Harriet Echo on July 19.*

1820   *Age thirty-five. Medical College of Ohio opens in fall; Drake is both president and professor of Institutes and Practice of Medicine. Founds the Western Museum Society housed in the Cincinnati College.*

1821   *Age thirty-six. January 16, Drake secures a state charter for the Commercial Hospital and Lunatic Asylum, the first hospital in United States primarily for teaching purposes and staffed exclusively by professors of a medical school.*

1822 *Age thirty-seven. March 7, Drake's colleagues vote to remove him as president and professor as a result of disagreements over direction of medical education. Plan for his treatise on the diseases of the western country is first identified in 1822 in the third number of* Godman's Western Quarterly Reporter.

1823 *Age thirty-eight. Assumes a professorship of medicine at Transylvania University. Eventually becomes dean of the faculty (November 1824–March 1827).*

1825 *Age forty. Wife Harriet Sisson Drake dies in Cincinnati on September 30 at the age of thirty-seven of "Autumnal Bilious Fever" (after eighteen years of marriage) before fall term at Transylvania University. Drake becomes a single parent with surviving children ages fourteen, eight, and six.*

✠ Beginning a Journal Editing Career

1827 *Age forty-two. Resigns from Transylvania University medical faculty, returns to Cincinnati, and joins with Dr. Guy W. Wright to establish and edit the* Western Medical and Physical Journal. *In April travels to Philadelphia to inspect the Eye Infirmary there and upon his return establishes the Cincinnati Eye Infirmary with special attention to eye care needs of the poor.*

1828 *Age forty-three. Starts a new medical journal as sole editor and publisher, the* Western Journal of the Medical and Physical Sciences, *with the dogwood bloom as emblem and the motto* E sylvis, aeque atque ad sylvas, nuncius *(Out of the forest, as well to the forest, the messenger). This journal is published continuously every month through June 1838; resumed in 1839 in Louisville as the* Western Journal of Medicine and Surgery. *Drake serves as editor through 1849. In September, Drake suffers severe burns to his hands while attempting to save, unsuccessfully, his sister-in-law, Caroline Sisson (age twenty) whose bed had caught on fire; Drake's hands are permanently scarred and he suffers severe depression and painful neuralgia that lasts for two years.*

1830 *Age forty-five. Accepts professorship (Theory and Practice of Medicine) at Jefferson Medical College in Philadelphia; lectures November through March. (Two volumes of his lectures for this year are archived at National Library of Medicine, Bethesda, MD.)*

✠ SECOND ATTEMPT TO START A MEDICAL SCHOOL IN CINCINNATI

1831   *Age forty-six. Returns to Cincinnati and initially seeks to form a new medical school with Miami University but is blocked by Medical College of Ohio faculty. He is asked to rejoin the faculty at the Medical College of Ohio, which he does for one year. Mother dies November 9, age seventy.*

1832   *Age forty-seven. Resigns from Medical College of Ohio after the 1831–1832 term. Publishes* A Practical Treatise on the History, Prevention, and Treatment of the Epidemic Cholera *in July. Cholera epidemic hits Cincinnati in September. Drake loses his father October 11 (age seventy-six) to cholera. Publishes* Practical Essays on Medical Education and the Medical Profession in the United States, *a landmark volume on how to improve the training of physicians.*

1833   *Age forty-eight. Advocates for a school for the instruction of the blind to be built in Ohio, near Columbus.*

1834   *Age forty-nine. Advocates for a system of national marine hospitals along the Ohio and Mississippi Rivers subsequently approved by 24th US Congress.*

1835   *Age fifty. Cincinnati College is restarted with William McGuffey as president; a medical department is created with Drake as dean. The Medical Department of Cincinnati College openly competes with the Medical College of Ohio with its first graduating class in 1836 and lasts for four years. It closes due to lack of funds and a hospital for teaching. Drake suffers repeated attacks by his competitors from the Medical College of Ohio.*

✠ BEGINNING PRIMARY RESEARCH WORK ON HIS SYSTEMATIC TREATISE

1836   *Age fifty-one. Once again Drake announces his plans for a book on the diseases of the Ohio Valley. At that time he realizes that "to travel as the only mode on which reliance can be placed [to gather data]. By visiting the principal localities on the great platform between the Great Lakes and the Gulf of Mexico, several important acquisitions can be made, either by direct personal observation, or by intercourse with gentlemen resident*

in different places" (Emmet Field Horine, Daniel Drake (1785–1852): Pioneer
Physician of the Midwest *[Philadelphia: University of Pennsylvania Press, 1961],
352). First travels May through the summer: Indiana, Illinois, Missouri, Alabama,
Tennessee, Kentucky, and back to Ohio.*

✠ A Decade at the Louisville Medical Institute

1839   *Age fifty-four. Many faculty resign from the Medical Department of Cincinnati College
due to closure of the Cincinnati Commercial Hospital to the medical faculty. The Medical
Department of Cincinnati College graduated 388 physicians in its four years of operation.*

    *Drake relocates to Louisville after accepting a position as professor of Clinical
Medicine and Pathological Anatomy at the Louisville Medical Institute in September
1839. On November 9 he delivers an introductory lecture.*

    *Drake continues to maintain his official residence in Cincinnati. During the aca-
demic sessions of the institute, he occupies an apartment in a college building at Eighth
and Chestnut Streets. During the winters in Louisville, he goes at least once a month on
weekends to visit both of his daughters who live in Cincinnati.*

    *Both daughters are married. Elizabeth (age twenty-two) marries Alexander
McGuffey, a lawyer and brother of the originator of the famous McGuffey readers.
Younger daughter Harriet Echo (age twenty) marries James Campbell, a business-
man and meatpacker.*

1840   *Age fifty-five. Drake is baptized in April at St. Paul's Church Episcopal Church in Louisville.*

1841   *Age fifty-six. Brother Benjamin dies, April 1 (age forty-six). He was a lawyer and
author in Cincinnati.*

1842   *Age fifty-seven. January, son Charles's wife, Martha Drake, dies. Continues with research
on his major work. Second trip, summer: the Great Lakes and their bordering states.*

1843   *Age fifty-eight. After the winter session in March 1843, Drake takes a third trip
traveling to New Orleans. During this trip he also travels to Pensacola, Florida, where
he tours the naval base. Visits the University of Alabama in Tuscaloosa.*

1844   *Age fifty-nine. Fourth trip, spring: he starts southward again and travels to Mobile, Alabama, and then returns to New Orleans. He continues traveling and visits Missouri, Illinois, and the upper reaches of the Mississippi River through October 1844. This summer journey covers 6,200 miles. Winter 1844 begins composition of the book.*

1845   *Age sixty. The vacation periods of 1845 and 1846 spent in Cincinnati continuing to write his book. "He was described as being methodical in all that he did, worked at a large table, which was covered with open books, journals from every section of the country, and embryonic manuscripts in every stage of development, from scraps of field notes, up to the perfected copy for the hands of the publisher" (Horine,* Daniel Drake, *358).*

1847   *Age sixty-two. Fifth trip, summer: West Virginia, Pennsylvania, western New York, and on to Quebec, Montreal, and Toronto in Canada. He returns to Louisville in November 1847.*

December 1847–January 1848, Drake writes a series of letters to his children describing his boyhood in Kentucky, later edited by his son Charles and published in 1870 as Pioneer Life in Kentucky: A Series of Reminiscential Letters to His Children.

1848   *Age sixty-three. In May a granddaughter (age fifteen months; son Charles's daughter) dies. Attends 2nd AMA Convention in Baltimore.*

⊠ Final Years in Louisville and Cincinnati

1849   *Age sixty-four. In March he resigns his professorship in Louisville due to nearing age of retirement and returns to the Medical College of Ohio to be closer to both daughters and grandchildren, and because his magnum opus was to be printed in Cincinnati. Printing completed in April 1850. Cholera returns to Cincinnati early 1849, and he loses a grandson, Joseph Charles Drake (age twelve) and James P. Campbell (age forty-three), Harriet's husband, to the disease.*

Resumes professorship at the Medical College of Ohio in Cincinnati in November. Attends 3rd AMA Convention in Boston and gives an opening session discourse on medical education.

1850   *Age sixty-five. Drake resigns from the Medical College after the AMA Convention and returns to the University of Louisville to teach for the next two academic years,*

1850–1851 and 1851–1852. Publishes Systematic Treatise, Historical, Etiological, and Practical, on the Principal Diseases of the Interior Valley of North America, *volume 1.*

The AMA meeting for 1850 was held in Cincinnati. At the convention Drake was lauded for his book on the Diseases of the Mississippi Valley *and he wept at this ovation.*

Summer of 1850 spent in Cincinnati busily engaged in writing second volume of his Diseases of the Mississippi Valley.

Drake becomes very interested in the slavery issue and the problems created by the Fugitive Slave Act.

1851   *Age sixty-six. In January, writes a letter to the Ohio State Convention on slavery. In April "Letters on Slavery to John C. Warren of Boston" were published. Drake attends the AMA meeting in Charleston, South Carolina.*

Late in 1851 Drake "fathers" the Cincinnati Medical Library Association, giving more than one hundred volumes as a nucleus of the collection.

1852   *Age sixty-seven. Drake opens the Medical Library's reading rooms by giving two addresses. The first on January 9 is entitled "Early Physicians, Scenery, and Society in Cincinnati." The second discourse January 10 is on "The Origin and Influence of Medical Periodical Literature and the Benefits of Public Medical Libraries."*

In early 1852 Drake resigns his professorship in the medical department of University of Louisville to accept position at the Medical College of Ohio in Cincinnati.

Drake returns once again to Cincinnati to begin the fall lectures. On the evening of October 26, Drake suffers severe, protracted chills. After a two-week illness he dies on Friday, November 5. The funeral was on Wednesday, November 10, in Cincinnati at Christ Church. He was then buried next to his wife in Spring Grove Cemetery in Cincinnati.

1854   *Volume 2 of his unfinished* Systematic Treatise, Historical, Etiological, and Practical, on the Principal Diseases of the Interior Valley of North America *is published posthumously.*

Acknowledgments

This book has had a long gestation period, with many direct and indirect contributors along the way.

The idea for the book originated as I was working on another book, *Becoming a Master Physician* (yet to be published). *Becoming a Master Physician* is similar in approach, using selections from the writings of many physician authors over different generations to help define the art of medicine and the journey to mastery as a physician. Working on that project introduced me to the writings of Daniel Drake, and in turn, to the Henry R. Winkler Center for the History of the Health Professions, the special collections library of the Donald Harrison Health Sciences Library at the University of Cincinnati College of Medicine Library. Billie Broaddus, former Health Sciences librarian and director of the Cincinnati Medical Heritage Center (forerunner of the Winkler Center), gave me my first book by Drake and helped me find other materials in the collection. When Billie retired in 2003 she was succeeded by Doris Haag. Both shared a deep passion for the center and Daniel Drake, and I thank them for their invaluable assistance.

I also wish to thank Dr. Jack McDonough, then chair of the Winkler Center Advisory Board, who invited me to join the board in 2010. As the University of Cincinnati was beginning to plan for the 2019 Bicentennial in 2012, Jack solicited ideas from the Advisory Board for ways to contribute to the celebration. Jack was very enthusiastic about the concept of this new work of Drake and shared it with the main bicentennial oversight committee. I began to work on the book in my spare moments, but Jack subsequently shared that the bicentennial subcommittees were being reorganized and the health committee was going to be merged with another committee. Then silence on whether the book had support to go forward, and I slowed down working on the book, and eventually stopped.

But then in May 2016 Dr. Ryan Hays, executive vice president from the President's Office, called me inquiring about the book proposal. What was it about? After a brief explanation Ryan suggested I should meet with Buck Niehoff (co-chair of the Spirit of History Committee, former member of the UC Board of Trustees, and visionary for the new UC Press) and Bob Dodds (then co-chair of the Bicentennial Committee) to explain the proposal. I owe much to these three individuals and appreciate their support of the project when all I had was a proposal and a few brief selections. They expressed faith in me to carry it forward, and without their support at that critical juncture and after, this book would not have been published.

I began to research and write in earnest about the same time that the University of Cincinnati (UC) Press was created. The UC Press, headed by Elizabeth Scarpelli and her staff of Sarah Muncy, Daniel Mattox, and Daniel Paul, have been incredible partners in this work. Liz's experience and expertise are evident in shaping the concept, providing guidance with early drafts, securing reviewers, working with the copy and design editors, and shepherding it through to final production. Liz, words cannot adequately express my gratitude to you for your thoughtful approach and wisdom. You clearly saw what the finished work could become before I could. Daniel, thank you for reading through the manuscript and helping shape the introduction. Sarah, thank you for the work behind the scenes—the known and unknown. Copyeditor Marilyn Campbell offered her skills and expertise with attention to detail, insightful edits, and recommendations and vastly improved the book. I am infinitely grateful for her help. Thank you, too, to the anonymous reviewers of the book who provided excellent feedback, critique, and offered suggestions on how to make the book better.

Staff from Special Collection Libraries have been essential to this work. I have mentioned already the staff members of the Winkler Center who were involved in getting me started, but I would be remiss if I did not mention those who were so helpful to me when I picked up the book again. Thank you to Leslie Schick and Lori Harris for enthusiastic encouragement and assistance in securing information from the National Library of Medicine. Thank you, too, to Veronica Buchanan who directed the creation of the Drake finding aid, assisted me with my questions, and secured the Drake resources I needed during her time there. Many thanks to Gino Pasi, the current archivist of the Winkler Center, who welcomed my intrusions, helped refine the Drake finding aid, and provided whatever I sought—a scanned picture, a book, or a journal.

I also wish to thank the staff at the University of Kentucky Health Sciences Library, and the King Library that houses its special collections. Thank you for assisting me with the Drake primary resources in the Emmet Field Horine Papers, and particularly Drake's *Verse Album*. Thank you too, to the National

LEAVING A LEGACY

Library of Medicine that provided a digital copy of Drake's *Common Place Book* from 1805 to 1806.

I have also had the good fortune of the support of faculty in the Department of Family and Community Medicine, and also the three deans during the time the book was being prepared: Dr. Thomas Boat, Dr. William Ball, and Dr. Andrew Filak. All have allowed me the space and time to work on and complete the book while serving as department chair of Family and Community Medicine. Special thanks to my excellent administrative staff, Melia Warnsley (Family Medicine) and April Dostie (Dean's Office). You have helped me with my schedule and created the opportunities to balance all my other duties while completing the book.

Finally, I would like to thank my family who have listened to and supported me through this long process amid vacations, weekends, and long days away at the College of Medicine campus, the hospital, or primary care office. My dear wife, Linda, knows me so well and has helped me stay true to the task, shares her patient listening ear, and expresses her confidence in all my work. I appreciate your love and support. To our growing family of seven children and their respective spouses, thank you for your patience and esteem, and realize this book will offer some guidance on how to create your own legacies.

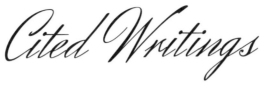

Cited Writings

of Daniel Drake

1. *Anniversary Address, Delivered to the School of Literature and the Arts at Cincinnati, November 23, 1814.* Cincinnati: Looker and Wallace, 1814.

2. *An Anniversary Discourse, On the State and Prospects of the Western Museum Society.* Cincinnati: Looker, Palmer, and Reynolds, 1820.

3. "Causes of Error in the Medical and Physical Sciences." In *Practical Essays on Medical Education and the Medical Profession in the United States.* Cincinnati: Roff & Young, 1832.

4. "Cincinnati Eye Infirmary." *National Republican and Ohio Political Register* 5 (November 16, 1827).

5. Committee on Defects in the Organization and Administration of Medical Schools. *Journal of the Proceedings of the Medical Convention of Ohio, at Its Second Session, Columbus, Ohio, January 1, 1838.* Cincinnati: 1838.

6. "Compensation of Physicians." *Western Journal of the Medical and Physical Sciences* 12 (1838): 49–56.

7. "The Description of the Buckeye." In *The Akron Offering: A Ladies' Literary Magazine, 1849–1850,* edited by Jon Miller. Akron, OH: University of Akron Press Publications, 2013.

8. "Discipline: Discourse on the Philosophy of Family, School, and College Discipline." *Transactions of the Fourth Annual Meeting of the Western Literary Institute and College of Professional Teachers.* [Meeting held in Cincinnati, October 1834.] Cincinnati: Josiah Drake Publisher, 1835.

9. "Early Physicians, Scenery, and Society of Cincinnati." In *Discourses Delivered by Appointment before the Cincinnati Medical Library Association.* Cincinnati: Moore and Anderson, 1852.

10. "Editorial: Clerical Encouragement of Quackery." *Western Journal of Medicine and Surgery* 4 (1841): 235–236.

11. "Editorial: Progress of Science." *Western Journal of Medicine and Surgery* 4 (1841): 403–404.

12. "Elements of Pathology." *Western Journal of the Medical and Physical Sciences* 11 (1838): 642–643.

13. "Emotions, Reflections, and Anticipations" [1826 or 1827]. In *Pioneer Life in Kentucky: A Series of Reminiscential Letters from Daniel Drake, M.D., of Cincinnati to His Children*, edited by Charles D. Drake. Cincinnati: Robert Clarke & Co., 1870.

14. "Epidemic Cholera." *Western Journal of the Medical and Physical Sciences* 7 (1833): 161–181.

15. "The Formation of Professional Character" [1835]. In *Frontiersman of the Mind*, edited by Charles D. Aring. Cincinnati: History of the Health Sciences Library and Museum, University of Cincinnati, 1985.

16. "History of Two Cases of Burn, Producing Serious Constitutional Irritation." *Western Journal of the Medical and Physical Sciences* 4 (1830): 48–60.

17. *An Inaugural Discourse on Medical Education.* [Delivered at the Opening of the Medical College of Ohio in Cincinnati, November 11, 1820.] Cincinnati: Looker, Palmer, and Reynolds, 1820.

18. *An Introductory Lecture, at the Opening of the Thirtieth Session of the Medical College of Ohio.* Cincinnati: Morgan and Overend, Printers, 1849.

19. "Lectures on Mental Philosophy of Students of Medicine." *Western Journal of the Medical and Physical Sciences* 10 (1836): 324.

20. "Legislative Enactments." In *Practical Essays on Medical Education and the Medical Profession in the United States.* Cincinnati: Roff & Young, 1832.

21. Letters. Cited in *The Life of Daniel Drake*, by Edward Mansfield. Cincinnati: Applegate & Co., 1855.

22. "Letters on Slavery to John C. Warren of Boston." The *National Intelligencer* [Washington, DC], April 3, 5, and 7, 1851.

23. "Lunatic Asylums." *Western Journal of Medicine and Surgery* 1 (1840): 380–384.

24. "Medical Colleges." In *Practical Essays on Medical Education and the Medical Profession in the United States.* Cincinnati: Roff & Young, 1832.

25. *Medical Diary; or, Common Place Book.* HMD Collection, 2931123R. National Library of Medicine, Bethesda, MD.

26. "Medical Hoax." *Western Journal of Western Journal of Medicine and Surgery* 3 (1841): 399.

27. "Memoir of the Miami Country 1779–1794" [an unfinished manuscript for the Western Historical Society]. *Quarterly Publication of the Historical and Philosophical Society of Ohio* 18 (1923): 2–3.

28. "A Memoir on the Diseases Called by the People 'Trembles,' and the 'Sick-Stomach' or 'Milk-Sickness'; as They Have Occurred in the Counties of Fayette, Madison, Clark, and Green in the State of Ohio." *Western Journal of Western Journal of Medicine and Surgery* 3 (1841): 176–179.

29. *A Narrative of the Rise and Fall of the Medical College of Ohio*. Cincinnati: Looker & Reynolds, Printers, 1822.

30. *Natural and Statistical View; or, Picture of Cincinnati and the Miami Country*. Cincinnati: Looker and Wallace, 1815.

31. "Neglect of Vaccination—Free Schools." *Western Journal of the Medical and Physical Sciences* 7 (1833): 156.

32. *The Northern Lakes: A Summer Residence for Invalids of the South*. Louisville, KY: J. Maxwell Jr., 1842.

33. *Notices Concerning Cincinnati*. Cincinnati: John W. Browne and Co., 1810.

34. "Observations and the Modus Operandi and Effects of Medicines." *Western Journal of the Medical and Physical Sciences* 1 (1827): 249–263.

35. "Observations on Some of the Uses and Abuses of Purgatives." *Western Journal of the Medical and Physical Sciences* 7 (1833): 32–42.

36. *Ohio Laws: Acts of the General Assembly*. Vol. 17. Chillicothe: George Nashee, 1819.

37. *An Oration on the Causes, Evils, and Preventives of Intemperance*. Columbus: Olmstead & Bailhache, Printers, 1831.

38. "The People's Doctors; a Review by 'The People's Friend.'{hrs}" *Western Journal of the Medical and Physical Sciences* 3 (1829): 393–420, 455–462.

39. *Pioneer Life in Kentucky: A Series of Reminiscential Letters from Daniel Drake, M.D., of Cincinnati to His Children*. Edited by Charles Drake. Cincinnati: Robert Clark & Co., 1870.

40. *Practical Essays on Medical Education and the Medical Profession in the United States*. 1832; Reprint, Baltimore: The Johns Hopkins University Press, 1952.

41. *A Practical Treatise on the History, Prevention, and Treatment of Epidemic Cholera, Designed Both for the Profession and the People*. Cincinnati: Cory and Fairbank, 1832.

42. "Private Pupilage." In *Practical Essays on Medical Education in the Medical Profession in the United States*. Cincinnati: Roff & Young, 1832.

43. "The Presidency I & II." *Liberty Hall & Cincinnati Gazette*, April 20 and 27, 1824.

44. *Railroad from the Banks of the Ohio River to the Tide Waters of the Carolinas and Georgia*. Cincinnati: Printed by James & Gazlay 1835.

45. "Professional Quarrels." In *Practical Essays on Medical Education and the Medical Profession in the United States*. Cincinnati: Roff & Young, 1832.

46. "Reform of the Medical College of Ohio." *Western Journal of the Medical and Physical Sciences* 9 (1835): 169–203.

47. "Remarks on the Importance of Promoting Literary and Social Concert, in the Valley of the Mississippi as a Means of Elevating Its Character and Perpetuating the Union." *Louisville: Members of the Convention at the Office of the Louisville Herald*, 1833.

48. "Report on the Necessity for Hospitals in the Valleys of the Mississippi and the Lakes for the Medical Convention of Ohio." *Western Journal of the Medical and Physical Sciences* 8 (1834): 461–462.

49. "School for the Instruction of the Blind." *Western Journal of the Medical and Physical Sciences* 7 (1833): 483–485.

50. "Selection and Preparatory Education of Pupils." In *Practical Essays on Medical Education and the Medical Profession in the United States.* Cincinnati: Roff & Young, 1832.

51. "Studies, Duties, and Interests of Young Physicians." In *Practical Essays on Medical Education and the Medical Profession in the United States.* Cincinnati: Roff & Young, 1832.

52. "Study of General and Pathological Anatomy." *Western Journal of the Medical and Physical Sciences* 9 (1835): 371–372.

53. *Systematic Treatise, Historical, Etiological, and Practical, on the Principal Diseases of the Interior Valley of North America as They Appear in the Caucasian, African, Indian, and Esquimaux Varieties of Its Population.* 2 vols. Cincinnati: Winthrop B. Smith & Co., 1850–1852.

54. "To the Physicians of the Western States." *Western Journal of the Medical and Physical Sciences* 2 (1828): i–vi.

55. "Traveling Editorials." *Western Journal of the Medical and Physical Sciences* 7 (1843): 239–240.

56. "Valedictory Address to the Class at Lexington in the Transylvania University, 1818." Daniel Drake Collection, Box 2, Folder 1. Henry R. Winkler Center for the History of the Health Professions, Donald Harrison Health Sciences Library, University of Cincinnati.

57. Verse Album of Daniel Drake, 1830–1836. Emmet Field Horine Papers (67M149), 1788–1863, Box 20, Folder 1. King Library, University of Kentucky Special Collections.

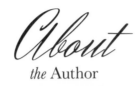

the Author

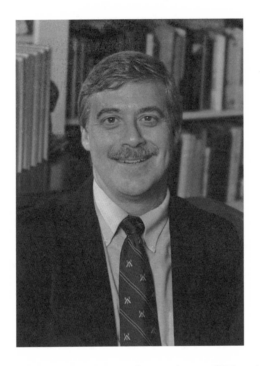

Philip M. Diller grew up in a small town in northwest Ohio where his father was a family physician and his mother an art teacher. He attended the College of Wooster (BA) and the University of Chicago (MD, PhD in Pathology). He completed his residency training in family medicine at the University of Cincinnati and has been on faculty at the UC College of Medicine since 1991. He served as Chair of the Department of Family and Community before assuming his current role as Senior Associate Dean for Educational Affairs. He practiced community family medicine for 23 years and now practices hospital palliative care medicine. He is an award-winning teacher who received the Exemplary Teacher of the Year in 2006 from the American Academy of Family Physicians. An avid medical historian, he serves as Chair of the UC Henry R. Winkler Center for the History of the Health Professions.